Multiple Choice Questions
PSYCHIATRY

Modern Nursing Series

General Editors

Susan E. Norman, SRN, NDN Cert, RNT, Senior Tutor, Nightingale School, West Lambeth Health Authority.

Jean Heath, BA, SRN, SCM, Cert Ed, National Health Learning Resources Unit, Sheffield City Polytechnic.

Consultant Editor

A. J. Harding Rains, MS, FRCS, Regional Dean, British Postgraduate Medical Federation; formerly Professor of Surgery, Charing Cross Hospital Medical School, University of London; Honorary Consultant Surgeon, Charing Cross Hospital; Honorary Consultant Surgeon to the Army

---

This Series caters for the needs of a wide range of nursing, medical and ancillary professions. Some of the titles are given below, but a complete list is available from the Publisher.

Multiple Choice Questions
Medicine, Surgery and Nursing
R. J. Harrison

Revision Notes on Psychiatry
K. T. Koshy

Psychology and Psychiatry
P. J. Dally

Community Child Health
M. E. Jepson

Nursing—Image or Reality?
Margaret C. Schurr
Janet Turner

Gerontology and Geriatric Nursing
Sir W. Ferguson Anderson
F. I. Caird
R. D. Kennedy
Doris Schwartz

Multiple Choice Questions and Answers:

PSYCHIATRY

Mary J. Watkins, SRN, RMN

Clinical Teacher in Psychiatry,
Nightingale School, West Lambeth Health Authority

HODDER AND STOUGHTON

LONDON SYDNEY AUCKLAND TORONTO

British Library Cataloguing in Publication Data

Watkins, Mary J.
  Multiple choice questions and answers:
  psychiatry.
  1. Psychiatry—Problems, exercises, etc
  I. Title
  616.89'0024613   RC457

  ISBN 0 340 28707 1

First published 1983

Printed in Great Britain for
Hodder and Stoughton Educational,
a division of Hodder and Stoughton Limited,
Mill Road, Dunton Green, Sevenoaks, Kent
by Biddles Ltd, Guildford, Surrey
Photoset by Rowland Phototypesetting Ltd,
Bury St Edmunds, Suffolk

Foreword

The questions in this book are close to the heart of psychiatric nursing and, when she makes her choices, the student nurse cannot help learning as well as using her knowledge. She is also likely to enjoy working through the items; she will get the answers right quite often and will find that some of the choices offered are fun as well as sharpening her perception of patients in their predicament.

Practice and feedback are essential for the development of skills and there is no doubt that in using this book the reader will develop a facility in answering multiple choice questions, not least in learning to attend closely to the wording of each one. When the question is one of what 'fits best' it may not be 'the truth' that will provide the right answer.

What fits best is, of course, a matter of judgement—in this case the author's, who in her answer section sets out the issues which have influenced her decision. It may be less apparent that the choice of validation procedures is dependent on judgement also; ultimately the new entrant to the profession must show that her judgement coincides to a large degree with that of established professionals.

Mary Watkins has done this profession a service not only by helping student nurses to refine their judgement but also in the cheerful and down to earth manner in which she has written this book.

Gunna Dietrich, BA, SRN, RMN, RNT
Senior Tutor, The Bethlem Royal
Hospital and The Maudsley Hospital
School of Nursing

Preface

This book is primarily aimed at psychiatric nurses studying for their final multiple choice question paper. It is intended to be a revision tool, so that when the student attempts the questions in the nursing section, she has revised psychology, psychiatry, communication and drugs.

Some of the questions are easier than others to motivate the student, and complicated questions have explanations attached to their answers. The questions have not been validated because the book aims to teach students as they work through it, but the 1982 Psychiatric Student Nurse syllabus has been the philosophy behind the book. The General Nursing Council (82/38) document setting out guidelines on Multiple Choice Questions has been considered and where appropriate questions have been compiled in this manner.

It is hoped that learner nurses will practice validated question papers in their schools of nursing, this book being designed as an additional instrument for them to use in private study. Some general learners will also find it constructive when undergoing a psychiatric secondment.

Mary Watkins

Contents

1 Psychology Questions

Concepts of Psychology

1 Which of the following is the best definition of psychology?

   (a) the study and understanding of normal mental functions and behaviour
   (b) the study and understanding of abnormal mental functions and behaviour
   (c) mental processes and physiological studies
   (d) the science of the physiological studies of the central nervous system

2 Which one of the following best describes the behavioural approach to the study of psychology?

   (a) interpreting man's feelings and emotions
   (b) studying man's emotions by observing them
   (c) observing man's behaviour
   (d) discussing man's behaviour

3 Which one of the following best describes the cognitive approach in the study of psychology?

   (a) man's physical, mental and biological development in relation to the environment
   (b) that the environment controls man's behaviour and that he is a passive receptor
   (c) that man is not a passive receptor but actively processes information and transforms it into relevant new forms
   (d) that man receives new forms of behaviour and behaves according to this

4 Which of the following best describes the psychological theory
   Freud developed?

   (a) that an individual is free to choose his own actions
   (b) the psychoanalytical concept, based on man's behaviour re-
        sulting from innate instincts that are largely unconscious
   (c) that certain unconscious processes result in biochemical
        change
   (d) that biochemical change in childhood causes damage to
        psychological development

Developmental Psychology

1 Which of the following is most helpful in contributing to language
   acquisition in children? To:

   (a) hear people speaking frequently
   (b) be spoken to by adults
   (c) hear adults converse and to be spoken to by them
   (d) be taught formally in a classroom

2 Who was the psychologist who stated that there are certain levels
   of development in children, one of which is the sensori-motor
   stage?

   (a) Freud
   (b) Binet
   (c) Skinner
   (d) Piaget

3 At which of the following ages does he say the sensori-motor stage
   occurs?

   (a) 0–2 years
   (b) 2–4 years
   (c) 4–6 years
   (d) 6–8 years

4 Which of the following best describes the changes taking place in
   adolescence?

   (a) biological, physical and sociological changes
   (b) biological and psychological changes
   (c) biological, physical and psychological changes
   (d) biological, psychological and sociological changes

5 Work helps a person to:

  (a) gain independence
  (b) gain social standing
  (c) gain ego identity
  (d) all of these

6 Which of the following is the clearest indication of maturity occurring in an individual?

  (a) selfishness
  (b) concern for others
  (c) getting married
  (d) having a baby

Intelligence

1 Which of the following best describes the meaning of intelligence?

  (a) intelligence is innate and does not relate to the environment
  (b) intelligence is the ability to adapt and learn
  (c) intelligence is the ability of man to adapt to the environment
  (d) intelligence is the product of experience and education

2 What is the best description of 'mental age'?

  (a) the measure of ability a person has reached
  (b) the ability a person should have reached
  (c) the age at which intellectualization is reached
  (d) the age at which one ceases to increase performance

3 Which of the following describes best the measure of time one has lived?

  (a) mental age
  (b) chronological age
  (c) actual age
  (d) old age

4 Intelligence quotient means which of the following?

(a) $\dfrac{\text{mental age}}{\text{chronological age}} \times 100$

(b) $\dfrac{\text{age}}{\text{mental age}} \times 100$

(c) $\dfrac{\text{chronological age}}{\text{age}} \times 100$

(d) $\dfrac{\text{chronological age}}{\text{mental age}} \times 100$

5 What is the normal range of IQs?

(a)   70– 85
(b)   85–110
(c)   85–115
(d)   115–130

6 What percentage of the population falls within the normal range of IQs?

(a) just above 70%
(b) 70%
(c) just under 70%
(d) 60%

7 At approximately 30 years of age which one of the following begins to decline on intelligence testing?

(a) the performance score
(b) the verbal score
(c) the verbal score if male and performance if female
(d) the performance score if male and the verbal if female

8 Which of the following statements is true with regard to intelligence? The more:

(a) unintelligent the person the slower the decline
(b) intelligent the person the slower the decline
(c) unintelligent the person the faster the decline
(d) intelligent the person the faster the decline

9 Many factors will affect performance in intelligence testing. Which of the following is least likely to affect the testing?

(a) hunger
(b) sex of the testee
(c) education
(d) anxiety

10 The term 'ability tests' includes aptitude and achievement tests. Which of the following best describes achievement tests?

(a) they measure what a person knows
(b) they measure accomplished skills and indicate what one can do at present
(c) they measure what a person could do if taught
(d) they measure what a person has learnt

Personality

1 Personality can be defined as the individual's characteristics and behaviour that, in their organisation, account for an individual's unique adjustments to his:

(a) family
(b) total environment
(c) occupation
(d) culture

2 Which of the following theories assumes that personality differences result from variations in learning experiences?

(a) the trait theory
(b) the psychoanalytic theory
(c) the social learning theory
(d) the humanistic theory

3 Freud saw personality as composed of three major systems. Which one did he say was present in the newborn infant?

(a) the *id*
(b) the *ego*
(c) the *superego*
(d) none of these

4 Freud stated that the id seeks pleasure, the ego tests reality and the superego strives for:

    (a) satisfaction
    (b) equilibrium
    (c) perfection
    (d) punishment

5 Which of the following is a personality test?

    (a) Wechsler Intelligence Scales
    (b) Stanford–Binet Test
    (c) Serial 7s
    (d) Minnesota Multiple Personality Inventory

6

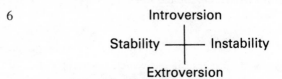

Which of the following personality theories assumes that a personality can be described by its position on a number of continuous dimensions, similar to those depicted above?

    (a) humanistic
    (b) trait
    (c) psychoanalytic
    (d) social learning

7 Which of the following are parts of an individual's personality?

    (a) behaviour and age
    (b) height and age
    (c) behaviour and thinking
    (d) thinking and height

8 How is a reserved, rather unsociable person described?

    (a) an extrovert
    (b) an introvert
    (c) stable
    (d) unstable

9 Which of the following has based a theory of personality on the dimensions introvert–extrovert and stable–unstable?

(a) Eysenck
(b) Jung
(c) Rogers
(d) Freud

10 A person who is an extrovert is most likely to seek employment as a:

(a) gardener
(b) salesman
(c) lighthouse man
(d) shepherd

Emotion

1 Which of the following is the best description of emotion? Emotion is a mental reaction to a stimulus which:

(a) may or may not be accompanied by physiological change
(b) must be accompanied by physiological change
(c) must not be accompanied by physiological or psychological change
(d) must be accompanied by physiological or psychological change

2 Which of the following would be the most difficult to measure accurately when taking measurements of changes which occur in anxiety?

(a) blood pressure and pulse
(b) pulse and sweating
(c) pulse and respiration
(d) blood pressure and respiration

3 Which of the following is most likely to occur if a person is very angry?

(a) a drop in temperature and pulse
(b) a drop in pulse and blood pressure
(c) a rise in pulse and blood pressure
(d) a rise in blood pressure and pulse

4 Which of the following neurological structures are involved in the control of emotions?

(a) medulla
(b) hypothalamus
(c) pons
(d) cerebellum

5 Which of the following are the two parts that make up the autonomic nervous system?

(a) reactive and sympathetic
(b) sympathetic and parasympathetic
(c) sympathetic and unreactive
(d) autonomic and sympathetic

6 Which of the following best describes what occurs in the body when intense emotion occurs? Arousal of the:

(a) autonomic system
(b) parasympathetic system
(c) sympathetic system
(d) reactive system

7 Activation of the sympathetic system results in a decrease in gastro-intestinal mobility. As a result, blood is diverted elsewhere. Blood is normally diverted to:

(a) smooth muscle and the central nervous system
(b) smooth muscle and the liver
(c) skeletal muscle and the central nervous system
(d) skeletal muscle and the liver

8 Which of the following is most likely to occur as a result of sympathetic activation during intense emotion?

(a) raised pulse and blood pressure, and pupil dilation
(b) raised pulse and blood pressure, and pupil contraction
(c) decreased pulse and blood pressure, and pupil contraction
(d) decreased pulse and blood pressure, and pupil dilation.

9 Which of the following is the best answer to the question 'Are emotions innate or learnt?'

(a) learning is important in modifying emotions but some forms appear to be innate
(b) emotions are entirely innate and develop through maturation
(c) emotions are entirely gained by experience
(d) emotions are not learnt but are probably innate, their expression is learnt by experience

10 Which of the following best describes the type of emotional arousal which can improve performance at a task?

(a) low levels
(b) high levels
(c) intense bursts
(d) prolonged intense levels

11 Which of the following terms describes 'stress illness' which can result from continual emotional tension?

(a) physiological illnesses
(b) psychoneurotic illnesses
(c) psychosomatic illnesses
(d) psychosexual illnesses

Motivation

1 Who was the famous psychologist who developed a hierarchy of motives ascending from basic biological needs to more complex psychological motives?

(a) Freud
(b) Skinner
(c) Maslow
(d) Jung

2 This hierarchy is often pictured as a:

(a) square
(b) pyramid
(c) circle
(d) rectangle

3 The first stratum of the hierarchy consists of which of the following?

 (a) cognitive needs
 (b) esteem needs
 (c) safety needs
 (d) physiological needs

4 The highest stratum of needs in the hierarchy is:

 (a) physiological
 (b) esteem
 (c) self actualisation
 (d) safety

5 Which of the following statements best describes the theory of this hierarchy?

 (a) a person is motivated to achieve all the needs at once
 (b) until a person has achieved the basic needs he cannot be motivated to achieve higher needs
 (c) the needs which a person is motivated to achieve depend on his intelligence
 (d) as a person matures he will gradually be motivated to achieve all these needs

6 The psychoanalytical theory of motivation is based on two basic human motives—Which are they?

 (a) fear and sex
 (b) sex and aggression
 (c) aggression and anxiety
 (d) anxiety and fear

7 Social learning theory discusses human motivation. It is based on which of the following?

 (a) learning, cognitive processes and self reinforcement
 (b) self reinforcement, cognitive processes and sexual drive
 (c) sexual drive, cognitive processes and learning
 (d) learning, self reinforcement and sexual drive

8 If aggression is a learnt response, which of the following theories best describes it?

(a) social learning theory
(b) psychoanalytical theory
(c) learning theory
(d) analytical theory

9 If aggression is described as an instinct or a frustration produced drive, which of the following theories best describes it?

(a) analytical theory
(b) innate theory
(c) psychoanalytical theory
(d) social learning theory

10 Which of the following best describes the factors most likely to motivate human behaviour?

(a) memory and biological drives
(b) biological drives and emotions
(c) emotions and intelligence
(d) intelligence and biological drives

Memory

1 Which of the following is the best definition of 'memory'?

(a) an unwritten record of past events that can be recalled
(b) an unwritten record of past events that can be recalled in response to relevant stimuli
(c) an ability to store information gained from earlier learning processes and reproduce it in response to relevant stimuli
(d) an ability to store an unwritten record of past events

2 Which of the following could be used as a mnemonic for this number—1066 1066?

(a) GOOD SHOW
(b) WELL WELL
(c) YOUR LOVE
(d) ONLY SOME

3 Which of the following is not likely to interfere with memory storage?

   (a) anxiety
   (b) hunger
   (c) gender
   (d) stress

4 Which of the following statements referring to memory have psychologists proved?

   (a) women have far more comprehensive memories than men
   (b) men have far more comprehensive memories than women
   (c) prolonged chemical and alcohol abuse affects long term memory more frequently than recent memory
   (d) prolonged chemical and alcohol abuse affects recent memory more frequently than long term memory

5 Which of the following places the three stages of memory in the correct order?

   (a) recognition, storage, retrieval
   (b) encoding, storage, retrieval
   (c) recognition, retrieval, storage
   (d) encoding, retrieval, storage

1 Psychology Answers

Concepts of Psychology

1 (a)
2 (c)
3 (c)
4 (b)

Developmental Psychology

1 (c)
2 (d)
3 (a)
4 (d)
5 (c)
6 (b)

Intelligence

1 (c)
2 (a)
3 (b)
4 (a)
5 (c)
6 (c)
7 (a) At the age of approximately 30 performances scores begin to drop; the more intelligent the person the slower the decline. Verbal scores may increase up to a higher age and then decline later than performance scores.
8 (b)
9 (b) Most adverse factors will affect performance, particularly sensory deprivation. Education may improve it.
10 (b) Achievement tests. Aptitude tests measure the capacity to learn and predict what a person could accomplish if educated to do so.

Personality

1 (b)
2 (c)
3 (a)
4 (c)
5 (d)
6 (b) A trait, refers to any characteristic in which one individual differs from another in a relatively permanent and consistent way.
7 (c) Personality is the *whole* person, his likes, dislikes, attitudes, moods and characteristic behaviour.
8 (b)
9 (a)

10 (b) An extrovert usually seeks the company of others. A salesman has to go out and seek others in order to sell his goods. The
other three occupations would be relatively quiet. (See Reference
below.)

Emotion

1 (a) There is generally a psychological change but not always.
2 (b) Sweating is the most difficult.
3 (c)
4 (b)
5 (b)
6 (c)
7 (c)
8 (a)
9 (d) (a) is also a good answer but not as detailed as (d).
10 (a)
11 (c)

Motivation

1 (c)
2 (b)
3 (d)
4 (c)
5 (b) (see Reference below)
6 (b)
7 (a)
8 (a)
9 (c)
10 (b)

Memory

1 (c)
2 (b) $W = 1, E = 0, L = 6$.
3 (c) All the others can affect perception.
4 (d) All the other statements are currently believed.
5 (b)

Reference
Hilgard, E., Atkinson, R. and R. (1983) *Introduction to Psychology* 7th edn. New York: Harcourt Brace Jovanovich Inc.

2 Communication Questions

1 Verbal communication can be varied in a number of ways. Which of the following is the most successful method with psychotic patients?

    (a) raising one's voice
    (b) lowering one's voice
    (c) speaking slowly
    (d) speaking slowly and concisely

2 Trust has to be built up in a relationship for effective communication. Which of the following is the best description of trust as a human value?

    (a) to feel someone cares
    (b) to feel someone cares and that they are reliable
    (c) to rely on someone
    (d) to feel someone is unquestionably reliant

3 Which of the following types of communication are most likely to build a relationship of trust with an anxious patient?

    (a) concise, direct, simple
    (b) honest, concise, efficient
    (c) honest, concise, practical
    (d) relevant, honest, clear

4 Non-verbal communication refers to 'body language'. Which of the following organs is most important in such communication?

    (a) hands
    (b) mouth
    (c) eyes
    (d) face

5 Which of the following is most likely to influence body language?
A person's

(a) height
(b) hair
(c) weight
(d) culture

6 Which of the following would be the best nursing approach if a
nurse wants a patient who is sitting down to feel that she cares
about him and has time to talk?

(a) to come up to him, stand opposite him and say 'Hello'
(b) to sit next to him crossing her arms and smiling
(c) to sit next to him, lean forward and attempt to make eye
contact
(d) to sit next to him with a relaxed posture and say 'Hello'

7 Which of the following would be the best approach to a depressed patient who finds eye contact nearly impossible? He does
talk reasonably well when relaxed.

(a) talk to him looking at the floor
(b) involve him in a task such as washing up
(c) sit opposite him
(d) watch television with him

8 A client in a group has been severely criticised by another and she
rests her head on her hand. Is this most likely to be a sign of

(a) boredom?
(b) regression?
(c) a self-supportive mechanism?
(d) frustration?

9 Is a 40 year old lady who is sitting on her bed, with her arms
folded, her head leaning forward, and rocking gently likely to be:

(a) happy?
(b) withdrawn?
(c) suicidal?
(d) manic?

10 How long is eye contact held between two people in 'normal' conversation?

   (a) 1 second
   (b) 5 seconds
   (c) 10 seconds
   (d) 1 minute

11 Sister is sitting in the office compiling the off duty rota. She doesn't like to be disturbed at this time. A first year student nurse is worried about a patient who is crying. She approaches the office for some help slowly and hesitantly. Why is this?

   (a) her low status
   (b) her fear of being reprimanded
   (c) her thought that possibly the patient is alright and therefore maybe she need not bother Sister
   (d) anxiety is high on the ward

12 Who has the highest status on an average psychiatric ward? The

   (a) doctor
   (b) sister
   (c) domestic
   (d) patient

13 In a therapeutic community who should have the most status?

   (a) the doctor
   (b) the patient
   (c) everyone
   (d) the domestic

14 How should a nurse ideally seat four patients when having a small discussion? In:

   (a) a straight line
   (b) a square
   (c) an informal circle/oval
   (d) a rigid circle

15 What does the term personal space mean in relation to an individual patient on a ward?

(a) eighteen inches around a person
(b) the small environment that is his own, e.g., his bed area
(c) where he sits at meals
(d) his own home

16 Which of the following describes best what the others are likely to do if a group leader uncrosses her legs?

(a) consciously follow suit
(b) not notice consciously
(c) unconsciously follow suit
(d) consider that the leader has uncrossed her legs

17 Why is it important if there are three people talking not to sit in a straight line?

(a) the middle person finds conversation hard
(b) the middle person may only talk to one person either side of her
(c) the middle person finds conversation hard and may only talk to one person
(d) confusion easily arises

18 A relative comes into the ward and demands to see the nurse in charge. He then complains about the ward saying that no one cares about his wife and that the hospital is disgusting. His wife was admitted the previous day on a Section 4 in a very neglected state. Is he most likely to be:

(a) angry with the nurses
(b) angry with his wife
(c) angry with himself
(d) feeling guilty

19 What is the most likely reason for a girl who took an overdose of drugs after a row with her boyfriend refusing to see him when he visits?

(a) she is not clean and tidy
(b) she feels guilty
(c) she is not sure she wants to go back to him
(d) she has been very distressed and really doesn't know what she wants

20 Which of the following best describes the term 'counselling', which is commonly used in nursing today?

    (a) advising the patient of avenues open to him
    (b) directing the client into what to do to help himself
    (c) showing the client avenues open to him and helping him to decide for himself what he wants to do
    (d) showing the patient avenues open to him and helping him to decide for himself what he wants to do

21 Which of the following is the best definition of feedback?

    (a) a process of checking out if the message sent is the message received
    (b) a process of checking out if the message sent is the message received and vice versa
    (c) a dynamic process of evaluation
    (d) the process of evaluation and understanding

22 The term 'listening' implies which of the following:

    (a) a passive act of taking in the content of another's conversation
    (b) an active process of responding to total messages
    (c) listening with one's ears and observing body language
    (d) (b) and (c)

23 Which of the following statements is true?

    (a) listening is a simple task
    (b) listening is innate
    (c) listening is a skill which can be effectively taught
    (d) personality does not affect listening skills

24 The term 'points' in body language refers to:

    (a) movements of the head, face and hands
    (b) movements of all limbs
    (c) movements of individual digits
    (d) facial movements

25 Which of the following is the most likely reason for a young man who is suffering from claustrophobia suddenly getting up and terminating a conversation?

(a) discomfort
(b) anxiety
(c) boredom
(d) anger

26 A patient cuts her wrists on a ward and is bleeding profusely. A senior nurse asks a junior nurse to telephone the doctor and ask him to come immediately. The junior nurse returns and says that the doctor is in a ward meeting and will come in twenty minutes. What is the most likely reason for the incompetence of the nurse's communication with the doctor?

(a) the junior nurse's anxiety and fear at the situation
(b) the senior nurse's inefficiency at not ensuring that the junior nurse clearly understood the reasons for the presence of a doctor
(c) the doctor's reluctance to come
(d) the doctor's anxiety at having to leave a meeting

27 What should the senior nurse do to ensure that the situation in question 26 does not arise again?

(a) leave the junior nurse and telephone herself
(b) ensure by the use of feedback that the nurse will give an accurate message
(c) take the patient to the office while she telephones the doctor
(d) complain to the consultant about the reluctance of the doctor to come to the ward

28 Which of the following would be the best nursing action if a patient who is generally very undemanding asks if he can speak to a nurse alone? The nurse is about to do the drug round.

(a) ask him if he can wait half an hour
(b) ask him how long it will take him to speak to you
(c) explain that if he would like a proper discussion it would be more convenient to speak to him after doing the drugs, but that if it is urgent you will see him immediately
(d) point out that she is is busy but that at some time in the day she will see him

29 Who of the following would be the best interpreter if a Polish
   woman who speaks no English is admitted to the ward? Her
   husband accompanies her but she keeps spitting at him and
   appears to be very angry with him.

   (a) her husband
   (b) another Polish patient who speaks English
   (c) a Polish priest
   (d) her daughter

30 What should the senior nurse do first if a student nurse comes into
   the office and bursts into tears?

   (a) tell her to pull herself together
   (b) sit her down and get her a cup of tea
   (c) establish that no one has physically hurt her on the ward
   (d) ask her to tell you her problem immediately as you are busy

31 Which of the following emotions is most likely to block effective
   communication?

   (a) mild anxiety
   (b) severe anxiety
   (c) moderate anxiety
   (d) continuous anxiety

32 Which of the following is least likely to block effective communication?

   (a) alienation
   (b) a feeling of belonging
   (c) interaction consciousness
   (d) a feeling of self-consciousness

33 Which of the following actions is most likely to be effective if a
   nurse wants someone to remember what she has said?

   (a) the nurse repeats what she has said
   (b) the nurse repeats what she has said and writes it down
   (c) the other person repeats what the nurse has said
   (d) the other person writes down what was said while the nurse
       repeats it

34 'I'm so frightened', says Mrs Brown. Nurse Smith replies 'So frightened'. Of which of the following is Nurse Smith's remark an example?

(a) postural echoing
(b) echoing
(c) a statement
(d) questioning

35 The following are examples of being both supportive and unsupportive in interaction with a client who is sitting down:
   1 sitting leaning forward to the speaker
   2 smiling
   3 standing up   4 rubbing one's face.
Which of the following would be most supportive?

(a) 1 and 2
(b) 2 and 3
(c) 3 and 4
(d) 4 and 1

36

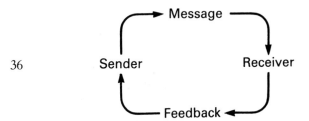

The diagram above is a model of

(a) feedback
(b) communication
(c) interaction
(d) understanding

37 It appears that a patient is about to throw a flower pot across the room. A nurse calls 'Mr Smith, put the flower pot down'. She could call 'What are you doing, tell me immediately?'

For which of the following reasons is the first remark most valuable in this situation?

(a) she says Mr Smith's name so that he knows she is speaking to him
(b) she is clear and concise about what she wants him to do
(c) she is clear, concise and states his name
(d) a command is always responded to more quickly than a question

38 Which of the following is the best way of allocating nurses if a suicidal patient is to be specialed?

(a) get all the staff to talk to him and share the burden
(b) allocate a nurse for the morning to sit and chat
(c) make a different nurse sit for one hour at a time, rotating two nurses
(d) sit the most senior nurse with him all morning

39 Which of the following would be the best way of handling a conversation in which the client suddenly becomes silent having been talking happily for five minutes?

(a) terminate the conversation
(b) sit quietly focusing attention on the client
(c) explain that if she does not talk it is difficult to help her
(d) ask her why she is not talking

40 In a well run ward which of the following is the most unlikely reason for a new nurse feeling anxious about communicating with the patients?

(a) the nurse's anxiety that she may say the wrong thing
(b) the nurse's anxiety of being reprimanded if she is not seen chatting to the patients
(c) the nurse's anxiety that the patients will not talk to her
(d) a fear on the nurses part that she may talk too much and not give the patients a chance to speak

2 Communication Answers

1 (d)

2 (b) There is a component of feeling that the person cares, in order to believe that they are reliable.

3 (d) Clarity is important when a patient is anxious. Without honesty trust has no firm foundation. The patient will respect and trust if relevant material is discussed.

4 (c) (see reference [1] below)

5 (d)

6 (d) (c) is too intense.

7 (b) (a) is modelling badly, (c) is too intense, (d) television can block conversation very easily.

8 (c) The patient is most likely to be giving self support but if she has no interest in the group it may be boredom.

9 (b)

10 (a)

11 (a) At no time did the question state (d). Both (b) and (c) relate to status.

12 (a)

13 (c)

14 (c) This is not a large enough group to warrant a rigid circle. Communication can be held effectively in a small informal circle.

15 (b)

16 (c)

17 (c)

18 (d)

19 (d) It could be any of the answers but the most likely reason is that she is not sure what she wants.

20 (c) It is imperative that the nurse does not perceive the person she is helping in the dependent role of patient but in the role of 'client'.

21 (b) Feedback is two way.

22 (d)

23 (c)

24 (a)

25 (b)

26 (b)

27 (b)

28 (c) 'A patient who is generally very undemanding'—these are the key words in the question.

29 (c) You may wish to ask her confidential questions which it would be inappropriate for her daughter to interpret.

30 (c) If violence has occurred this may need to be dealt with immediately. Then you can do (b). (d) would produce an answer but unless it was something tangible on the ward she may feel unable to discuss it after such an approach.

31 (b) Is the most likely.

32 (b)

33 (d)

34 (c) There is no question mark.

35 (a)

36 (b)

37 (c)

38 (c) Such interaction is very anxiety provoking. If nurses stay for more than an hour their observation skills decline. You must make *one* person responsible at a time so that the patient is adequately supervised and that each nurse does not think another is observing him.

39 (b) This will show her you are interested and give her time to collect her thoughts. (a) would be very rejecting. (c) and (d) are rather demanding but may be required if Mrs Brown continued to remain silent.

40 (b) If the ward is well run the senior nurse will have explained that no one expects her to make relationships with the patients immediately.

References

1 Argyle, Michael (1975) *Bodily Communication*. London: Methuen & Co.

2 Argyle, Michael (1981) *Social Skills and Health*. London: Methuen & Co.

3 Argyle, Michael (1978) *Social Interaction*. London: Tavistock

4 Argyle, M., and Trower, P. (1979) *Person to Person—Ways of Communication*. New York: Harper and Row.

3 Psychiatry Questions

Definitions

1 Hallucinations are examples of disorders of:

(a) affect
(b) perception
(c) volition
(d) thought

2 A perception of sensory vividness with no apparent external stimuli is:

(a) a delusion
(b) an illusion
(c) an hallucination
(d) a paranoia

3 Which of the following mental mechanisms is being used excessively by a patient suffering from hysterical paralysis?

(a) conversion
(b) projection
(c) denial
(d) dissociation

4 Regression can be most accurately described as:

(a) banishment of unacceptable wishes or ideas from conscious awareness
(b) turning of interests inwards to total pre-occupation with self
(c) unconscious efforts to erase a previous painful experience
(d) resumption of behaviour typical of an earlier level of development

5 Agoraphobia is fear of:

(a) open spaces
(b) high places
(c) being alone
(d) flying

General Psychiatry

1 Which of the following statements best defines the form of speech that consists of a string of disconnected words, with no logical form?

(a) word salad
(b) flight of speech
(c) knight's move
(d) thought blocking

2 Which of the following describes the symptom of a patient not feeling himself, but feeling 'cut off' from everything around him and unreal?

(a) derealisation
(b) disorientation
(c) depersonalisation
(d) dissociation

3 In which of the following illnesses is 'Flattening of Affect' most likely to be present?

(a) manic depressive psychosis
(b) Korsakov's psychosis
(c) schizophrenia
(d) reactive depression

4 Which of the following words best describes the misinterpretation of a real sensory stimulus?

(a) illusion
(b) hallucination
(c) delusion
(d) rationalisation

5 Which of the following mental mechanisms describes the process whereby a quality of another person is taken into and made a part of the subject's personality?

(a) impression
(b) projection
(c) introjection
(d) regression

6 Which of the following statements best describe the symptom of a young woman with schizophrenia who complains of an obnoxious smell, which you cannot smell at all?

(a) nihilistic delusion
(b) olfactory hallucination
(c) tactile hallucination
(d) visceral hallucination

7 A young girl of 14 years is admitted in an emaciated state with a diagnosis of anorexia nervosa. Which of the following is not a symptom of this illness?

(a) severe weight loss
(b) dysmenorrhoea
(c) amenorrhoea
(d) active refusal to eat

8 Which of the following observations would you carry out first on a patient receiving 200 mg Chlorphromazine a day, if she complained of feeling dizzy?

(a) temperature
(b) pulse
(c) pupil reaction
(d) blood pressure

9 The most appropriate description of an hysterical personality would be:

(a) episodes of rage and verbal and physical aggressiveness
(b) attention seeking, over reactive, emotionally labile
(c) low energy level, lack of enthusiasm, over sensitive to emotional stress
(d) responds to situations with ineptness and social instability

10 Which of the following drugs is most likely to cause addiction?

(a) Chlormethiazole
(b) Chlorpromazine
(c) Haloperidol
(d) Trifluoperazine

11 In the psychiatric field the drug dependent patient is most frequently associated with which of the following?

(a) personality disorder
(b) depression
(c) schizophrenia
(d) adolescence

12 A patient who displays the problem of cross dressing from male clothes to female clothes is called a:

(a) homosexual
(b) heterosexual
(c) transvestite
(d) paedophiliac

13 With which of the following diseases should a nurse wear gloves for her own protection when dealing with a patient who has scratched himself several times:

(a) Alzheimer's disease
(b) Parkinson's disease
(c) Jakob-Creutzfeldt syndrome
(d) Huntington's chorea

14 Which one of the following statements best defines the term 'Exogenous' which is used to describe a depressive illness?

(a) neurotic or psychotic
(b) neurotic or reactive
(c) psychotic or reactive
(d) endogenous or neurotic

15 When does involutional melancholia most frequently occur for the first time?

(a) youth
(b) early middle age
(c) late middle age
(d) old age

16 Which of the following types of personality describes a person who has regular mood swings from feeling happy to feeling sad?

(a) hysterical
(b) schizoid
(c) explosive
(d) cyclothymic

17 Which of the following statements best describes the term 'asthemic' in relation to personality?

(a) passive, dependant and negative
(b) volatile and attention seeking
(c) cautious, meticulous and inflexible
(d) sensitive and suspicious

18 Which of the following must be present in a young girl with anorexia nervosa?

(a) depression
(b) constipation
(c) amenorrhoea
(d) vomiting

19 Which of the following is most likely to be present in a patient suffering with hypomania?

(a) paranoid delusions
(b) delusions of grandeur
(c) delusions of poverty
(d) secondary delusions

20 A young girl of nine still suffers from nocturnal enuresis. Which of the following best describes this?

(a) incontinence
(b) bedwetting
(c) urinary incontinence at night
(d) double incontinence at night

21 Which of the following statements best describes the term 'delu-
    sion'?

(a) a firm, fixed, false belief, not related to culture
(b) a misconception of thought
(c) a misconception of sense
(d) a false belief that cannot be changed

22 From which of the following types of schizophrenia is a patient
    most likely to be suffering if he often displays suspicion about
    other patients?

(a) hebephrenic
(b) simple
(c) catatonic
(d) paranoid

The Functional Psychoses

1 Which of the following people first used the term schizophrenia?

(a) Emil Kraeplin
(b) Eugene Bleuler
(c) Sigmund Freud
(d) Kurt Schneider

2 The term 'functional psychosis' refers to:

(a) schizophrenia
(b) organic psychosis
(c) organic psychosis and schizophrenia
(d) manic depression and schizophrenia

3 The risk of developing schizophrenia in the general population is:

(a) 0.5%
(b) 1.0%
(c) 1.5%
(d) 2.0%

4 Which of the following statements best describes the reason for a person's work record being an important aid to diagnosis?

(a) it may show a person has not found the work he likes
(b) it often measures stability and perseverance
(c) it is an indication of perseverance and happiness
(d) it may reflect the unemployment situation

5 The term 'affect' can best be used to replace which of the following words?

(a) excitement
(b) perception
(c) mood
(d) volition

6 If a person describes how his father has recently died and giggles while doing this, is this most likely to be:

(a) flattening of affect
(b) splitting of affect
(c) incongruity of affect
(d) depersonalisation

7 Which of the following is most likely to be present in a patient with schizophrenia?

(a) tactile hallucinations
(b) auditory hallucinations
(c) visual hallucinations
(d) olfactory hallucinations

8 Which of the following is always present in an hallucinatory experience:

(a) a mental impression
(b) an external stimulus
(c) an auditory experience
(d) a visual experience

9 In which of the following groups of illness are visual hallucinations most common?

(a) functional psychosis
(b) acute organic psychosis
(c) dementias
(d) depressions

10 The schizophrenic may be unable to maintain his train of thought because of:

(a) thought blocking
(b) pressure of thought
(c) flight of ideas
(d) ideas of reference

Neuroses

1 Which of the following is the chief characteristic in neurotic disorders?

(a) fear
(b) anxiety
(c) unhappiness
(d) displacement

2 Which of the following is the best definition of 'neurosis'?

(a) emotional maladaptation due to conflict within societies
(b) emotional maladaptation due to conflict within families
(c) emotional maladaptation due to conflict within the personality
(d) emotional maladaptation due to conflict within relationships

3 Which of the following statements is most accurate regarding neurotic illness?

(a) thinking, judgement and contact with reality may be severely impaired
(b) thinking and judgement may be impaired with minimal loss of contact with reality
(c) thinking, judgement and contact with reality will be impaired
(d) thinking and judgement should be unimpaired, with minimal loss of contact with reality

4 Neurotic patients use ego defence mechanisms to reduce:

(a) fear
(b) unhappiness
(c) anxiety
(d) excitement

5 Which of the following sets of defence mechanisms are most commonly utilised by neurotic patients?

(a) displacement and projection
(b) displacement and regression
(c) denial and displacement
(d) displacement and conversion

6 Which of the following best describes the commonest cause of neurotic illness?
Interaction of a person's constitution and personality with his:

(a) family
(b) environment
(c) work situation
(d) financial situation

7 Which of the following sets of relationships is most likely to contribute to the development of neurotic illness?

(a) sibling
(b) parent–child
(c) female–male
(d) extended family

Dementia

1 Which of the following types of dementia is hereditary?

(a) Parkinson's disease
(b) Huntington's chorea
(c) Alzheimer's disease
(d) general paralysis of the insane

2 Which of the following symptoms is a patient diagnosed as having Korsakov syndrome likely to display?

   (a) generalised memory damage
   (b) no memory damage
   (c) damage to short term memory
   (d) damage to long term memory

3 Which of the following diseases most commonly causes dementia?

   (a) arteriosclerosis
   (b) severe bronchitis
   (c) glomerulonephritis
   (d) deep vein thrombosis

4 A 70 year old lady in your ward has a dementia, and her relatives have asked you how best to help her manage at home. Which of the following replies would be best?

   (a) label all plugs with the name of the implement to which they relate; change gas appliances for electric wherever possible and keep her mobile.
   (b) establish a simple fixed regime and routine
   (c) maintain mobility, but do everything possible for the lady; never leave her alone
   (d) maintain mobility while establishing a fixed regime and routine

5 Which one of the following statements referring to mobility allowance is correct? The claimant must be:

   (a) over 65
   (b) under 65
   (c) between the ages of 5 and 65
   (d) over 60 if female, 65 if male

6 Which of the following statements best describes the environment in which a lumbar puncture should be carried out? In a

   (a) sterile theatre
   (b) aseptic situation
   (c) clean bed
   (d) well ventilated room

7 For a diagnosis of pre-senile dementia to be made, the patient must be younger than:

(a) 50 years
(b) 60 years
(c) 79 years
(d) 80 years

8 When a person has contracted Huntington's chorea how long afterwards does death usually occur?

(a) 6–12 weeks
(b) 1–2 years
(c) 10–12 years
(d) this is not usually fatal

9 Which of the following defines the term 'Choreoathetoid movements' which are displayed in Huntington's chorea?'

(a) sinuous
(b) quick and jerky
(c) of the face
(d) Parkinsonian

Depression

1 The term 'mood' is often referred to as:

(a) effect
(b) affect
(c) personality
(d) anxiety

2 Is the patient with a depressive illness most likely to be:

(a) happy and responsive
(b) smiling and unresponsive
(c) gloomy and despondent
(d) withdrawn but content

3 Which of the following statements is true?

  (a) people who talk of suicide never kill themselves
  (b) only patients with endogenous depression commit suicide
  (c) people who suffer a variety of depressive illnesses commit suicide
  (d) only patients with reactive depression commit suicide

4 How many people in the United Kingdom are likely to develop some type of depressive illness?

  (a) 1 in 5
  (b) 1 in 10
  (c) 1 in 15
  (d) 1 in 20

5 The term 'reactive depression' implies that:

  (a) there is a strong precipitating factor
  (b) there is a strong genetic influence
  (c) external factors are of secondary importance
  (d) there is evidence of psychosis

6 Which of the following is the term given to the opposite type of depression to 'neurotic', using the same form of classification?

  (a) endogenous
  (b) reactive
  (c) unipolar
  (d) psychotic

Alcoholism

1 Which of the following statements is false?

  (a) there is increasing incidence of alcoholism
  (b) there is decreasing incidence of alcoholism
  (c) alcoholism has serious far reaching effects on society
  (d) alcoholism has serious effects on an alcoholic's family

2 Which of the following statements is not present in the World
  Health Organisation's definition of an alcoholic?

  (a) alcoholics drink beneficial amounts of alcohol
  (b) alcoholics have mental health or bodily problems
  (c) alcoholics' interpersonal relations become disturbed
  (d) alcoholics have difficulty functioning socially

3 Which of the following is the main reason for making alcoholism
  difficult to define?

  (a) some people can drink a bottle of whisky a day with no ill
      effects
  (b) not many people who drink heavily suffer physiological
      damage
  (c) taking alcohol in reasonable amounts is a socially accepted
      custom
  (d) some people drink too much because they want to

4 Does alcoholism occur:

  (a) only in men
  (b) only in people with low intelligence
  (c) predominantly in people with low intelligence
  (d) in all strata of society

5 Does an alcoholic tolerance for alcohol

  (a) remain static
  (b) decrease
  (c) progressively develop
  (d) develop, then decrease

6 How does an alcoholic present in the morning?

  (a) bright and cheerful
  (b) shaky and happy
  (c) nauseated and cheerful
  (d) nauseated and shaky

7 Which of the following is primarily affected in Korsakov's syndrome?

(a) sight
(b) liver
(c) memory
(d) heart

8 Do delirium tremens usually occur after abstinence of alcohol for:

(a) 12 hours
(b) 24 hours
(c) 2–3 days
(d) 4–7 days

9 Which of the following is a common mental complication of alcoholism?

(a) endogenous depression
(b) manic depressive psychosis
(c) paranoid states
(d) phobic anxiety states

Epilepsy

1 When is epilepsy first most likely to occur?

(a) childhood
(b) adolescence
(c) middle age
(d) old age

2 Which of the following statements best describes the symptoms of a patient who experiences an 'aura' in epilepsy?

(a) peculiar sensations
(b) peculiar smells
(c) peculiar tastes
(d) peculiar noises

3 In which of the following illnesses is computerised tomography brain scanning most likely to be helpful in aiding diagnosis?

(a) grand mal epilepsy
(b) cerebral tumours
(c) temporal lobe epilepsy
(d) petit mal epilepsy

4 A patient you are nursing suddenly falls to the floor, develops muscular ridgidity and stops breathing. Which of the following statements describes this part of an 'epileptic fit' most accurately?

(a) the tonic phase
(b) the clonic phase
(c) the tonic and clonic phases
(d) the total of a grand mal fit

5 Which one of the following best describes the term 'automatism'?

(a) a person's actions performed which are later not remembered
(b) a person takes on an automatic role
(c) a person is in a daze and will do anything they are asked
(d) a person is completely institutionalised

6 Which of the following types of epilepsy most frequently displays 'automatism'?

(a) grand mal
(b) Jacksonian seizure
(c) temporal lobe
(d) petit mal

7 Which of the following statements describes best the most serious complications of status epilepticus?

(a) repeated apnoea, which leads to too little carbon dioxide to the brain and an accumulation of oxygen
(b) lack of oxygen to the brain
(c) lack of oxygen to the limbs
(d) repeated apnoea, which leads to lack of oxygen to the brain and an accumulation of carbon dioxide

8 Which of the following observations should a nurse carry out prior to a patient having an electro-encephalogram for investigation into epilepsy? The doctor decides that in order to get an accurate reading the patient should not have any Phenobarbitone for 48 hours before the EEG. The patient has been taking it for 5 years.

(a) pupil reaction
(b) closely supervise him to ensure that if he fits he cannot hurt himself
(c) temperature, pulse and respiration
(d) pupil reaction and pulse

Day Hospital Care

1 Are day hospitals likely to:

(a) play an increasing role in the treatment available for the mentally ill
(b) play a decreasing role in the treatment available for the mentally ill
(c) continue to play a role in the treatment of the mentally ill at a stable level
(d) gradually run down and be replaced entirely by a community psychiatric nurse service

2 Day hospitals and day centres overlap in the services they offer. Which of the following is the major difference the services they are intended to provide?

(a) day hospitals should provide 'social aspects of care' while day centres provide 'medical aspects of care'
(b) day centres should provide 'social aspects of care' while day hospitals provide 'medical aspects of care'
(c) day centres should provide 'physical aspects of care' while day hospitals provide 'psychological aspects of care'
(d) day hospitals should provide 'physical aspects of care' while day centres provide 'psychological aspects of care'

3 The majority of those who use day hospitals live in:

(a) sheltered accommodation
(b) hospitals
(c) their own homes
(d) mental after care hostels

4 Lay hospitals for the mentally ill aim to serve people who present
with

(a) neurotic illness
(b) psychotic illness
(c) a full range of psychiatric illness
(d) mental illness and problems of mental impairment

Controversial Aspects of Psychiatry

1 Thomas Szasz says that the concept of mental illness is analogous
to:

(a) religion
(b) witchcraft
(c) alienation
(d) rejection

2 What is the general name for people who are in some way deviant
and are persecuted for their actions?

(a) schizophrenics
(b) sociopaths
(c) psychopaths
(d) scapegoats

3 Which statement is true regarding the following situation:
A patient is detained by the courts under Section 37 and a criminal
is convicted and sent to prison for the same crime.

(a) one is unquestionably mentally ill
(b) the criminal was aware of his crime but the patient was not
(c) the patient may be detained for an unlimited time, the criminal
serves a fixed penalty
(d) the criminal is punished but the patient is not

4 The term 'double binding' refers to a person who:

(a) verbally states one thing and nonverbally states the opposite
(b) nonverbally and verbally states the same thing
(c) raises his voice while reprimanding someone
(d) reinforces unacceptable behaviour

5 It has been suggested that schizophrenic illness can be potentiated
  by:

  (a) over-possessive mothers
  (b) over-possessive fathers
  (c) double binding mothers
  (d) double binding fathers

3 Psychiatry Answers

Definitions

1 (b) All the senses can be affected.
2 (c)
3 (a)
4 (d)
5 (a)

Reference
Dally, P. (1982) *Psychology and Psychiatry*. 5th edn. Sevenoaks:
  Hodder and Stoughton.

General Psychiatry

1 (a)
2 (c)
3 (c)
4 (a)
5 (c)
6 (b)
7 (c) This is painful periods.
8 (b) A drop in blood pressure is a common cause of dizziness
       when a patient takes Chlorpromazine.
9 (b)

10 (b)
11 (a)
12 (c)
13 (c) Recent reports say that this may be contagious, from blood of a patient.
14 (b) This is an illness that has an external precipitant.
15 (c)
16 (d)
17 (a)
18 (c)
19 (b) The others may be present.
20 (c)
21 (a)
22 (d)

Reference
Dally, P. (1982) *Psychology and Psychiatry*. 5th edn. Sevenoaks: Hodder and Stoughton.
Or
Sainsbury, M. J. (1980) *Key to Psychiatry*. London: H. M. & M. Publishers.

The Functional Psychoses

1 (b) in 1911.
2 (d)
3 (b)
4 (b)
5 (c)
6 (c)
7 (b)
8 (a) Hallucination can occur without a psychotic illness being present. There is a mental impression of sensory vividness, with no external stimuli.
9 (b)
10 (a)

Neuroses

1 (b)

2 (c)
3 (b)
4 (c)
5 (d)
6 (b)
7 (b)

Reference
Sainsbury, M. J. (1980) *Key to Psychiatry*. London: H. M. & M.
   Publishers.

Dementia

1 (b)
2 (c)
3 (a)
4 (d)
5 (c)
6 (b) This encompasses the others.
7 (b)
8 (c)
9 (b)

Depression

1 (b)
2 (c) Smiling depression is seen from time to time but is less
   common.
3 (d) The other statements are false.
4 (b)
5 (a) (b) and (c) apply mainly to endogenous depression. (d) this
   may be so but it is relatively uncommon.
6 (d)

Reference
Dally, P. (1982) *Psychology and Psychiatry*, 5th edn. Sevenoaks:
   Hodder and Stoughton.

Alcoholism

1 (b) Alcoholism is on the increase.
2 (a) Alcoholics do not drink beneficial amounts of alcohol.

3 (c) The main reason is that it is socially acceptable. Alcoholism is easier to define in Islamic cultures as drug addiction is in ours.
4 (d)
5 (d)
6 (d) Rarely do alcoholics feel cheerful in the morning.
7 (d) Short term memory is frequently lost.
8 (c)
9 (c)

Reference
Dally, P. (1982) *Psychology and Psychiatry,* 5th edn. Sevenoaks: Hodder and Stoughton.

Epilepsy

1 (a)
2 (a) Taste and smell most commonly.
3 (b) Rarely is epilepsy a space occupying lesion.
4 (a)
5 (a)
6 (c)
7 (d)
8 (b)

Day Hospital

1 (a) (see page 36)
2 (b) (see page 37)
3 (c) (see page 40)
4 (c) Provision is made for those with mental impairment separately unless they are suffering from a mental illness.

Reference
Wing, J. K. and Olsen, R. (1979) *Community Care for the Mentally Disabled.* Oxford University Press.

Controversial Aspects of Psychiatry

1 (b) (see Reference [1] below)
2 (d) (see Reference [1] below)
3 (c) A Section 37 can be terminated at the psychiatrist's wish. Thus the patient may serve a longer period than the criminal. (a), (b) and

(d) are all debatable. Enforced psychiatric care can be interpreted as punishment. (See Reference [2] below.)

4 (a) An example is a mother who is dressed up to go out and says to her child 'John, kiss Mummy goodnight'. When he slobbers on her make-up she freezes and pushes him away.

5 (c) Largely mothers as they generally spend more time with their children than fathers in Western Society.

References

[1] Szasz, T. (1971) *The Manufacture of Madness.* London: Routledge and Kegan Paul.

[2] Laing, R. D. and Esterson, O. (1970) *Sanity, Madness and the Family.* Harmondsworth: Penguin Books.

4 Drug Questions

1 Which of the following is the primary action of major tranquillisers?

(a) central nervous system stimulant
(b) central nervous system depressant
(c) autonomic nervous system stimulant
(d) autonomic nervous system depressant

2 Which of the following types of illness are most likely to respond
to minor tranquillisers?

(a) the neurotic disorders
(b) the psychotic disorders
(c) the behavioural disorders
(d) the depressive disorders

3 A section of the Misuse of Drugs Act 1973 refers specifically to
the major addictive drugs. These are known as controlled drugs.
These drugs must be kept under lock and key in a special
cupboard, preferably within another locked cupboard. Which of
the following statements indicates what else may be stored here?

(a) scheduled poisons
(b) intramuscular injections
(c) patients' valuables
(d) nothing at all

4 Which of the following are most likely to influence tolerance of
drugs?

(a) the sex and age of a patient
(b) the sex and weight of a patient
(c) the age and weight of a patient
(d) the weight and culture of a patient

5 A poisons centre exhibits in a major London teaching hospital. It is open 24 hours a day and can be telephoned for specific advice if an uncommon substance has been swallowed. If a nurse does not know which hospital this is, which of the following departments is most likely to have this information immediately at hand?

(a) administration
(b) nursing personnel
(c) accident and emergency
(d) theatres

6 The sun is shining brightly. Mr Brown who is 65 and takes Chlorpromazine 100 mg wants to sit outside. He is bald. Which of the following pieces of clothing is essential for him to wear?

(a) gloves
(b) a hat
(c) socks
(d) a neck scarf

7 A woman of 50 is put on Chlorpromazine. Two days later she complains of swollen breasts and lactation. Which of the following statements describes this?

(a) a very rare side effect of Chlorpromazine
(b) a side effect of Chlorpromazine
(c) a toxic effect of Chlorpromazine
(d) this probably bears no relation to Chlorpromazine

8 An old lady taking Chlorpromazine complains that she finds it difficult to read even with her glasses. Which of the following is the most likely explanation?

(a) she is developing cataracts
(b) she is anxious
(c) it is a toxic effect of Chlorpromazine
(d) because of her age her eyes need retesting

9 Which of the following side effects occurs most frequently with Haloperidol therapy?

(a) skin rashes
(b) blurred vision
(c) Parkinsonism
(d) jaundice

10 What should be the first action of a nurse who believes that a patient has taken a large dose of Chlorpromazine?

(a) try to induce vomiting
(b) telephone for medical assistance
(c) take his blood pressure
(d) ring for an ambulance

11 Which of the following side effects of psychiatric drugs can good nursing care normally prevent?

(a) constipation
(b) skin rashes
(c) diarrhoea
(d) urinary retention

12 In which of the following illnesses is Diazepam least likely to be used effectively?

(a) epilepsy
(b) anxiety neurosis
(c) schizophrenia
(d) agitated depression

13 Which of the following illnesses responds to Lithium salt treatment best?

(a) schizophrenia
(b) manic depressive psychosis
(c) thyrotoxicosis
(d) agitated depression

14 Which of the following drugs has recently been reported as causing potential dependence problems?

(a) Diazepam
(b) Chlormethiazole
(c) (a) and (b)
(d) Chlorpromazine

15 Which of the following drugs is not an anticonvulsant?

(a) Phenobarbitone
(b) Primidone
(c) Phenelzine
(d) Phenytoin sodium

16 Which of the following must a nurse do when administering a doze of Digoxin 0.25 mg to an elderly lady? Record her:

(a) pulse before administration
(b) pulse after administration
(c) blood pressure before administration
(d) blood pressure after administration

17 Which of the following should cause a nurse to omit a dose of Digoxin?

(a) a blood pressure of 120/80
(b) a pulse of 90
(c) a pulse of 56
(d) a blood pressure of 140/90

18 Which of the following salts may a patient need to supplement large doses of a diuretic?

(a) sodium chloride
(b) potassium chloride
(c) lithium carbonate
(d) sodium sulphate

19 Which of the following should be used to sterilise equipment required to mix young babies' feeds?

(a) Hibiscrub
(b) Ether
(c) Maxolon
(d) Milton

20 If a patient with tuberculosis was given the drug Rifampicin should the nurse warn him that:

(a) his urine may develop a red colouration
(b) his urine may develop a blue colouration
(c) he may develop severe constipation
(d) he may develop severe diarrhoea

21 A person who has been abusing barbiturate drugs is most likely to suffer from which of the following during rapid withdrawal?

(a) hallucinations
(b) delusions
(c) convulsions
(d) a rise in blood pressure

22 Penicillin may be prescribed 'before meals'. Is this because:

(a) the acidity of the stomach is at its lowest and the absorption is affected by conditions of acidity, thus maximum absorption is ensured

(b) the acidity of the stomach is at its highest and the absorption is affected by conditions of acidity, thus maximum absorption is ensured

(c) it may make a patient feel nauseated if taken after a meal

(d) none of these

23 The controlled drugs section of the Misuse of Drugs Act 1973 states that if a doctor requests a controlled drug:

(a) the ward sister or nurse concerned may give the doctor the keys of the Controlled Drugs cupboard

(b) the ward sister or nurse concerned will unlock the cupboard door and remain present

(c) that the doctor must be specially registered

(d) none of these

24 A dose of 0.5 mg of Atropine is required. The ampoules available contain 0.4 mg in 1 ml. The required dose will be:

(a) 1.1 ml

(b) 1.2 ml

(c) 1.25 ml

(d) 1.3 ml

25 A bottle of Methadone linctus is 20 mg in 5 ml. Your patient is prescribed 32 mg, how many millilitres will you give?

(a) 7 ml

(b) 8 ml

(c) 9 ml

(d) 10 ml

26 Which one of the following is the most dangerous toxic effect of monoamineoxidase inhibitor drugs when mixed with certain foodstuffs?

(a) a rise in pulse

(b) a drop in pulse

(c) a rise in blood pressure

(d) a drop in blood pressure

27 Which of the following foodstuffs is most dangerous with monoamineoxidase inhibitors?

(a) alcohol
(b) tyramine
(c) carbohydrates
(d) soluble fats

28 Which of the following drugs is not a phenothiazine?

(a) Phenelzine
(b) Chlorpromazine
(c) Stelazine
(d) Haloperidol

29 Which of the following drugs may not be used to counteract parkinsonism side effects of phenothiazines?

(a) Orphenadrine
(b) Benzhexol
(c) Diazepam
(d) Procyclidine

30 Which of the following illnesses is most likely to respond to oil based major tranquillisers intramuscularly?

(a) manic depressive psychosis
(b) schizophrenia
(c) phobic anxiety states
(d) psychotic depression

4 Drug Answers

1 (b)
2 (a)
3 (d)

 4 (c)
 5 (c)
 6 (b)
 7 (b)
 8 (d)
 9 (c)
10 (b)
11 (a)
12 (c)
13 (b)
14 (c)
15 (c)
16 (a)
17 (c)
18 (b)
19 (d) Hibiscrub and ether could kill a baby
20 (a)
21 (c)
22 (a)
23 (b)
24 (c)
25 (b)
26 (c)
27 (b)
28 (d)
29 (c)
30 (b)

5 Nursing Questions

Nursing Process

1 Is the main aim of the nursing process to provide

   (a) individualised care?
   (b) institutionalised care?
   (c) organised care?
   (d) psychological care?

2 Which of the following is the first stage of the nursing process?

   (a) planning
   (b) implementation
   (c) assessment
   (d) evaluation

3 If a plan of nursing care for a particular problem fails which of the following should the team do?

   (a) plan another method of care
   (b) re-assess the patient's problem
   (c) ask the patient for his opinion
   (d) re-assess the patient's problems with him

4 Which of the following should be written in an elderly patient's care plan if she only drinks tea? She needs to drink more.

   (a) get her to drink as much as possible
   (b) offer her drinks regularly, two litres/24 hours if possible
   (c) she likes tea. Try to increase her fluid intake to two litres/24 hours
   (d) encourage her to drink tea, she likes tea

5 Mrs Griffin is severely depressed. She has not expressed any suicidal ideas. Which one of the following would be the best plan of care for Mrs Griffin on an a.m. shift?

(a) student Nurse Jones to be responsible for Mrs Griffin
(b) ask all the nurses to be conscious of Mrs Griffin's whereabouts
(c) make sure that one nurse is responsible for any one part of the shift
(d) keep Mrs Griffin in her nightclothes

6 Which of the following are essential if the nursing process is to be implemented on a psychogeriatric ward of twenty patients?

(a) at least six nurses a shift
(b) four baths and six toilets
(c) personalised clothing for the patients
(d) at least three qualified nurses a shift

7 Which of the following lists the four stages of the 'nursing process' in the correct order?

(a) planning, assessment, implementation, evaulation
(b) assessment, planning, implementation, evaluation
(c) assessment, implementation, planning, evaluation
(d) implementation, assessment, planning, evaluation

8 Mrs O'Brien is forty years old. She is suffering from severe depression. She never speaks except when spoken to. The nursing team is feeling very despondent about her. Which of the following would it be best for the senior nurse to ask a student to do?
Please sit with Mrs O'Brien:

(a) this morning
(b) for at least half an hour
(c) for as long as you can manage
(d) for half an hour and then come and discuss it with me

9 Mr Bell has suffered from hypotension due to a reaction to Chlorpromazine. How would you write down the required nursing action?

(a) observe Mr Bell for hypotensive episodes
(b) take Mr Bell's blood pressure four hourly
(c) take and record Mr Bell's blood pressure four hourly and ask him if he feels dizzy when you do this
(d) explain to Mr Bell that he should inform a nurse if he feels dizzy. Take and record his blood pressure four hourly.

10 Miss Prior is very confused. The doctors have not found the cause for her confusion and ask you to observe her closely. Which of the following nurses would you ask to spend a morning with Miss Prior to obtain as accurate account as possible of her mental state?

(a) a nursing assistant
(b) a staff nurse
(c) a first year pupil nurse
(d) a first ward student nurse

Community Psychiatric Nursing

1 Which of the following is the main reason for the community psychiatric nurse having a different relationship with her patients from that of the psychiatric ward sister.

(a) the patients are less ill if at home
(b) the community nurse is a guest not a hostess
(c) the ward sister may be responsible for 'institutionalised' patients
(d) the community nurse sees her patient less frequently

2 Which of the following is the community psychiatric nurse most likely to be asked to visit?

(a) an identified patient
(b) a problem family
(c) a married couple
(d) a subnormal child

3 For which of the following reasons is a community psychiatric nurse least likely to be asked to visit a patient?

(a) to assess his mental state
(b) to assess his physical state
(c) regulating drug regimes
(d) communicating with a disturbed patient

4 If a patient is referred to a community psychiatric nurse which of the following would be the most legitimate reason?

(a) because the patient did not need to be seen by a psychiatrist
(b) because the general practitioner was too busy
(c) for distinct psychiatric nursing skills
(d) to relieve their families

5 In 1984 do the majority of community psychiatric services provide:

(a) a twenty-four hour on call system
(b) an 8.00 a.m., until 6.00 p.m., Monday to Friday service
(c) a crisis intervention team
(d) all of these

6 Community psychiatric nursing services first began in?

(a) the 1940s
(b) the 1950s
(c) the 1960s
(d) the 1970s

7 The World Health Organisation believes that:

(a) psychiatric nursing care should remain hospital based
(b) psychiatric nursing care should be equally hospital and community based
(c) it is of primary importance that the psychiatric nursing service is extended to the community
(d) psychiatric nurses should also do a general nurse training

8 With which of the following people is the community psychiatric nurse most likely to liaise?

(a) social workers and health visitors
(b) social workers and the clergy
(c) health visitors and the clergy
(d) clergy and the police

9 A community psychiatric nurse is likely to have a caseload of approximately:

(a) 25 people
(b) 35 people
(c) 45 people
(d) 55 people

10 Which of the following is the most valid reason for using the 'Nursing Process' in the community?

(a) concise record keeping
(b) it helps the nurse to set realistic goals
(c) it helps the nurse to work in a systematic manner
(d) it helps the nurse to work towards individualised patient care

11 When visiting Mr Sandeman, a 26 year old man with a phobic disorder, which of the following is the most important for the psychiatric nurse to ascertain, in addition to his personal characteristics and levels of functioning?

(a) Mr Sandeman's family's assessment of the patient
(b) Mr Sandeman's assessment of his problems
(c) the doctor's assessment of Mr Sandeman
(d) the social worker's assessment of Mr Sandeman

12 If a nurse were planning Mr Sandeman's care when should she arrange to review this with him?

(a) once a week
(b) as they go along
(c) at a predetermined date
(d) once a month

Nursing with Reference to Sociology and Roles

1 To be a competent psychiatric nurse it is necessary to have an understanding of the behavioural sciences. The three main behavioural sciences are:

  (a) sociology, psychology and physics
  (b) physics, psychology and anthropology
  (c) anthropology, sociology and psychology
  (d) sociology, anthropology and physics

2 The term 'role' is frequently used today. Which of the following is the subject of 'role theory'?

  (a) the job one has
  (b) human behaviour as displayed in social situations
  (c) the relationships a person has with his family
  (d) the relationships a person has in social situations

3 A patient is sometimes described as having taken 'the sick role'. Does this mean:

  (a) he is playing at being sick
  (b) his actions are relevant to those of a sick person
  (c) he has ceased to be a responsive adult
  (d) his behaviour has regressed

4 Do nurses' uniforms:

  (a) reinforce the 'role' of a nurse
  (b) inhibit the 'role' of a nurse
  (c) both reinforce and inhibit the 'role' of a nurse
  (d) not influence the 'role' of a nurse

5 If a patient is to undergo 'psychometric testing' which of the following people is most likely to do this?

  (a) the psychiatrist
  (b) the psychologist
  (c) the neurologist
  (d) the physiotherapist

6 In the rare event of a patient having a leucotomy, who will do this?

   (a) the psychiatrist
   (b) the neurologist
   (c) the neurosurgeon
   (d) the psychoanalyst

7 Is the difference between a psychologist and a psychiatrist that:

   (a) a psychiatrist is medically qualified and a psychologist is not
   (b) a psychologist is medically qualified and a psychiatrist is not
   (c) a psychiatrist cannot practise psychoanalysis and a psycholog-
        ist can
   (d) a psychologist cannot practise psychoanalysis and a psychiat-
        rist can

8 A psychiatric community nurse is asked to visit Mrs Weston, a 30
   year old lady, by her General Practitioner. Mrs Weston gave birth
   to a baby daughter sixteen weeks ago and has since become
   depressed. When visiting, the nurse becomes worried about the
   baby's feeding. Whom should she contact?

   (a) the community midwife
   (b) the district nurse
   (c) the health visitor
   (d) the social worker

Nursing Ethics

1 Which of the following best disproves the statement 'Behavioural
   treatment is an inhuman and degrading form of treatment'?

   (a) all behavioural treatments seek to give pleasure to patients
   (b) there are areas for which no alternative treatments are avail-
        able, not to attempt to give assistance is inhuman
   (c) drug treatments can be far more degrading and inhuman than
        behavioural treatments
   (d) electro-convulsive therapy is an equally inhuman and degrad-
        ing treatment

2 When planning behavioural therapy it may be necessary to give back to patients responsibility for their own behaviour. This may involve an element of risk. How best should this be monitored?

(a) by careful calculation based on the principles of behavioural treatment with official approval
(b) the patient should be asked only to do as much as he desires
(c) the patient should always be accompanied when leaving the hospital
(d) behavioural programmes should not be planned by student or pupil nurses

3 When should punishment techniques be used in behavioural nursing practice?

(a) never
(b) when no effective alternative method is available
(c) when a patient is physically aggressive
(d) in token economy schemes

4 Which of the following actions would be most appropriate if you become aware that a colleague is suffering from depression which is affecting her work. You have tried to discuss it with her but she insists there is nothing wrong.

(a) tell her senior nurse informally
(b) tell her that you must inform her senior nurse informally
(c) wait for two weeks to see how she manages
(d) tell her you will give her two weeks to sort herself out

5 Nurses give prime attention to administering safe care so that:

(a) the patient responds to treatment
(b) the patient receives good care
(c) the patient comes to no harm
(d) the patient maintains dignity

6 Which of the following is the most important for the nurse to recognise as a patient's right?

(a) to make his own decisions and be independent
(b) freedom of choice
(c) to refuse medication
(d) personal privacy

7 The Mental Health Act of 1983 states that it is illegal for which of the following:

(a) any nurse to have sexual intercourse with any patient
(b) a female nurse to have sexual intercourse with a male patient
(c) a male nurse to have sexual intercourse with a female patient
(d) nurses to have sexual intercourse with a patient of their own sex

8 Which of the following would be the best action to take if a patient says that he will only tell you something if you 'keep it to yourself':

(a) agree to this and keep it to yourself
(b) agree to this but then tell the other nursing staff
(c) point out that you cannot do this politely but firmly
(d) listen to him and then decide what to do

The Mental Health Act

1 When did the present Mental Health Act receive the Royal Assent?

(a) 1980
(b) 1981
(c) 1982
(d) 1983

2 When did the majority of the sections in the Mental Health Act become law? At the end of:

(a) August 1983
(b) September 1983
(c) October 1983
(d) November 1983

3 The new Mental Health Act:

(a) repeals the 1959 Mental Health Act
(b) replaces the 1959 Mental Health Act
(c) amends the 1959 Mental Health Act
(d) does not affect the 1959 Mental Health Act

4 Section 3 of the Mental Health Act 1983 initially detains patients for:

(a) three months
(b) six months
(c) nine months
(d) twelve months

5 The Act states that nurses qualified in the psychiatric field may contain a patient in the absence of a psychiatrist/doctor. Who are these nurses?

(a) Registered Mental Nurses
(b) Enrolled and Registered Mental Nurses
(c) Charge Nurse/Sisters (RMN)
(d) Nursing Officers (RMN)

6 The holding power that these nurses may use under the Act is for up to:

(a) two hours
(b) four hours
(c) six hours
(d) eight hours

7 The Act allowed for which of the following commissions to be set up?

(a) The Mental Welfare Commission
(b) The Mental Health Commission
(c) The Mentally Ill Commission
(d) The Mental Health Act Commission

8 The Commission set up by the Mental Health Act should include a large number of doctors and roughly equal numbers of:

(a) social workers, laymen, clergy, lawyers and nurses
(b) psychologists, social workers, laymen, clergy and lawyers
(c) nurses, psychologists, social workers, laymen and clergy
(d) lawyers, nurses, psychologists, social workers and laymen

9 For which of the following reasons can nurses detain a patient under Section 5 of the Mental Health Act 1983?

  (a) that it is not possible to secure the attention of a doctor
  (b) that the patient is suffering from mental disorder to a serious degree
  (c) that it is not practicable to secure the immediate attention of a doctor and the nurse believes the patient may harm himself or others if he leaves
  (d) when the nurse believes the patient may be a nuisance to his relatives and it is not practicable to secure the immediate attention of a doctor

10 When the Commission set up by the Act investigates a patient who is being treated without his consent, the members must consult which of the following about the patient?

  (a) his doctor, his psychologist and one other professional involved
  (b) his doctor, his social worker and one other professional involved
  (c) his doctor, his nurse and one other professional involved
  (d) his doctor, his occupational therapist and one other professional involved

Brenda Tewson—attempted suicide

A 22 year old girl is admitted to an acute admission ward at 6.00 p.m. She has been admitted from the Accident and Emergency Department of your local hospital. She has made several superficial cuts on her left wrist. She is clean and tidy but distressed because her boy friend has recently left her. She is an informal patient.

1 Which of the following facts would be the most important to determine after showing her around the ward

  (a) that her parents know her whereabouts
  (b) that she has nightclothes
  (c) that she has no sharp objects or pills in her possession
  (d) if she has had any supper

2 The ward has three single siderooms and four three bedded units. Which of the following would be the best place to put her for the night if the only beds available are

(a) in the side room near the office
(b) in a side room well away from the office
(c) in a unit with two elderly ladies
(d) in a unit near the office with one other woman

3 Which of the following would be the best nursing action if, after showing her which is to be her bed, she sits down on it and begins to cry.

(a) to say that you will leave her alone until she feels like talking
(b) stand opposite her and ask her what the matter is
(c) sit down beside her and show that you are willing to listen
(d) sit and offer her reassurance saying 'everything will be alright'

4 At 10.00 p.m., she says that she is worried because her flatmate doesn't know where she is. She is much calmer. Which of the following would be the best way of informing her flatmate?

(a) the nurse ringing the flatmate
(b) getting the patient to phone her flatmate
(c) asking the doctor to telephone her flatmate
(d) leaving it until the morning

Electro-convulsive Therapy

1 Before taking a patient to electro-convulsive therapy the nurse should ensure that the patient has emptied his bladder because

(a) he may be feeling anxious and have stress incontinence
(b) he may be incontinent during his fit if his bladder is full
(c) he may wish to pass urine directly after his treatment when he should be resting
(d) this is routine before an anaesthetic

2 How long should a patient be starved before electro-convulsive therapy?

(a) as directed by the doctor
(b) four hours
(c) six hours
(d) eight hours

3 Who must ensure that a voluntary patient has consented to electro-convulsive therapy, prior to treatment?

(a) the accompanying nurse
(b) the psychiatrist
(c) the anaesthetist
(d) all of these

4 The nurse's role while a patient is having electro-convulsive treatment is to:

(a) ensure he maintains an airway
(b) ensure that he fits properly
(c) ensure that he doesn't hurt himself
(d) ensure that his colour is satisfactory

5 Which of the following is most important when the nurse is observing a patient during the recovery stage after electro-convulsive therapy treatment?

(a) that the patient is warm enough
(b) that the patient's airway is maintained
(c) that the patient's pulse does not exceed 90 beats per minute
(d) to observe the blood pressure closely

6 Which of the following apparatus must the nurse place by the bed of a patient during the initial recovery stages after ECT?

(a) oxygen
(b) a suction apparatus
(c) a cardiac monitor
(d) a padded spoon

7 Which of the following statements describes the best nursing management post-ECT, assuming some patients like to sleep, others to have something to eat?

(a) assess the patient's individual needs
(b) ensure each patient has a warm drink
(c) allow any patient to have a rest if necessary
(d) give a patient whatever they want to eat

Mr Morgan—confusion

Mr Morgan is a 55 year old man who has been admitted in a confused state. He has a history of alcohol abuse. He has been suspended from duty at the Bank where he has been a clerk for twenty years. Recently he has become forgetful and seems to have trouble adding up long lists of figures. He lives alone.

1 Which of the following actions should be given priority?

(a) detoxification from alcohol
(b) psychometric testing
(c) plenty of rest and good food
(d) electro-encephalogram

2 After three days Mr Morgan still has trouble remembering the nurses' names, but remembers his own birthday and the year he was born. Which part of his memory appears to be damaged?

(a) sensory register
(b) recent memory
(c) long term memory
(d) memory recall

3 He may be prescribed Parentrovite High Potency Injections by the medical staff. Which vitamins does Parentrovite contain?

(a) vitamin A and B vitamins
(b) B vitamins and vitamin C
(c) vitamin C and D
(d) vitamin D and B vitamins

4 The Doctors diagnose his illness as an 'alcoholic dementia'. Which
   of the following will it be?

   (a) Alzheimer's disease
   (b) Korsakov syndrome
   (c) depressive psychosis
   (d) Pick's disease

Mr Meredith—confusion

An 82 year old man called Mr Meredith has been admitted in a
confused state. He has evidently not taken care of his hygiene or
nutrition for several days. His 60 year old daughter accompanied
him.

1 From whom would you try to gain a nursing assessment?

   (a) the daughter
   (b) Mr Meredith
   (c) Mr Meredith and his daughter
   (d) Mr Meredith, his daughter and your own observation

2 Having obtained a history which of the following would be your
   first concern?

   (a) to see that he has a wash
   (b) to see that he has a drink
   (c) to see that he has some food
   (d) to see that he has a good rest

3 Which of the following statements best describes how this patient
   should be nursed?

   (a) primary care
   (b) applying the nursing process
   (c) individualised nursing care
   (d) team allocation

4 Which of the following nursing actions is most likely to reduce Mr
   Meredith's confusion?

   (a) an adequate diet
   (b) group therapy
   (c) a course of phenothiazines
   (d) individual psychotherapy

5 Mr Meredith expresses considerable anxiety about having a bath, saying 'No young girl is going to bath me'. He says that he generally just has a good wash at home. Which of the following statements describes the most appropriate nursing action?

(a) agree for him to wash his face and hands
(b) insist that he has a bath and arrange for a male nurse to accompany him
(c) reassure him explaining you often help the gentlemen to bath
(d) ask for a male nurse to try and get Mr Meredith to have a strip wash

Diabetes

1 A patient with diabetes is given insulin to:

(a) raise his blood glucose level
(b) reduce his blood glucose level
(c) raise his blood sugar level
(d) reduce his blood sugar level

2 Which of the following methods is most commonly used to give insulin to a patient suffering from diabetes?

(a) oral
(b) intramuscular
(c) subcutaneous
(d) intravenous

3 A diabetic patient complains of thirst and his breath smells. On testing his urine, both glucose and ketones are present. Which of the following is he most likely to be suffering from?

(a) too much insulin
(b) too little insulin
(c) dehydration
(d) starvation

4 Which of the following actions should a nurse take if, after giving him his dose of insulin the patient feels drowsy and begins to sweat profusely.

(a) get him to lie down and rest
(b) take his temperature, pulse and blood pressure
(c) inform the doctor
(d) give him 50 g of glucose in a glass of water

5 Which of the following is the normal range of blood glucose level?

(a) 5–7 moles/litre
(b) 5–7 millimoles/litre
(c) 7–11 moles/litre
(d) 7–11 millimoles/litre

Mrs Jones—agitated depression

A forty year old housewife called Mrs Jones has been admitted to the ward with a diagnosis of agitated depression. Her daughter has just got married and left home. This is her first psychiatric illness.

1 Which of the following is the most likely cause of her illness, given the above information?

(a) marital disharmony
(b) the menopause
(c) that her daughter has left home
(d) that she has lost her previous role as her daughter has married and left home

2 Where would Mrs Jones best be placed in the ward?

(a) in a single room
(b) in a double room with a patient with paranoid schizophrenia
(c) in a small bay with two ladies also suffering from depression
(d) with an elderly lady with dementia

3 Which of the following would be the most important action for the nurse to take on Mrs Jones' admission?

(a) to take her clothes away and get her to sign for them
(b) to get her husband's telephone number
(c) to introduce her to some other people on the ward
(d) to explain that you are a nurse and that if there is anything she doesn't understand to ask you

4 What action should the nurse take if when admitting Mrs Jones she finds she has a large pair of dressmaking scissors?

(a) ask her husband to take them home
(b) establish if needlework is one of her hobbies and if so let her keep them
(c) explain that they can be kept in the office and she could have them when she needs them
(d) explain that she could borrow the ward scissors when necessary and her husband could take the others home

5 At her first meal on the ward Mrs Jones says she doesn't want anything to eat. Which of the following describes the best method of dealing with this?

(a) insisting she eats
(b) telling her it's up to her and you don't mind what she does
(c) seeing if there is anything she would like, for example a hot drink
(d) pointing out that this is a hospital and she ought to conform

Miscellaneous

1 Which of the following illnesses is a common complication of alcoholism?

(a) thyrotoxicosis
(b) anorexia nervosa
(c) liver cirrhosis
(d) ulcerative colitis

2 Day care is becoming increasingly successful in the care of psychiatric patients. Which of the following statements about day care is not true in relation to hospital care?

    (a) a patient is less likely to become institutionalised
    (b) a patient is less likely to become regressed
    (c) a patient can be more easily observed
    (d) a patient is more likely to keep his role in society

3 What is the most important reason for allowing patients to keep some of their own small possessions around them in hospital?

    (a) it contributes to their sense of security and belongingness
    (b) it helps to orientate them
    (c) it increases their motivation to get better to go home
    (d) it reminds them of when they were well

4 When a patient is suffering delirium tremens, which of the following is the nurse likely to observe?

    (a) raised temperature, raised blood pressure and raised pulse
    (b) raised temperature, lowered blood pressure and raised pulse
    (c) lowered temperature, raised blood pressure and raised pulse
    (d) raised temperature, lowered blood pressure and lowered pulse

5 When writing a nursing report on the patient which of the following should the nurse do?

    (a) ensure that she initials it
    (b) state the time, date and sign it
    (c) clearly state the date and sign it
    (d) ensure that the report is illegible

6 Which of the following would be the most appropriate method of helping an elderly man who is having increasing difficulty with eating meals. He continually drops food down his shirt, due to poor co-ordination.

    (a) give him a bib
    (b) give him a large napkin
    (c) feed him
    (d) give him a liquid diet

7 A lady of 68 has been transferred from an orthopaedic ward having recently fractured her femur. She is depressed and withdrawn. The medical staff request that she should be up, dressed and mobilised. When helping her in the bathroom a nurse slips and they both fall down. Which of the following would the senior nurse wish to ensure, having first established that neither was hurt?

(a) that the nurse was taking reasonable care
(b) that the nurse was acting according to policy
(c) that the nurse was taking reasonable care and acting according to policy
(d) that the lady is never taken to the bathroom without two nurses again

8 Which of the following is most likely to influence the standards of nursing care on the ward?

(a) attitudes of the medical staff
(b) attitudes of the nursing staff
(c) attitudes of patients
(d) availability of nursing aids, e.g. hoists

Anne Leak—weight loss

A thirteen year old girl called Anne with a history of severe rapid weight loss and apathy is admitted to an acute psychiatric ward where behavioural techniques are sometimes used in treatment.

1 Which of the following is the most likely diagnosis of Anne's problems?

(a) schizophrenia
(b) adolescent crisis
(c) anorexia nervosa
(d) depression

2 For a diagnosis of anorexia nervosa to be made which of the following is not true?

(a) the patient must be female
(b) at least 10% of body weight must be lost
(c) no signs of organic disease must be found
(d) there must be an active refusal to eat

3 Which of the following words describes the phrase 'Determined, sustained efforts to prevent ingested food from being absorbed'?

(a) vomiting
(b) bulimia
(c) gastritis
(d) reflex vomiting

4 If Anne is to be treated by behaviour modification techniques. Which of the following is the best way to begin her nursing care?

(a) allow her freedom on the ward
(b) strict bedrest
(c) bedrest but up for washing and toileting
(d) ask Anne what she wants to do

5 If Anne is placed on a behaviour therapy programme, which of the following would be the best method of weighing her in the initial stages of treatment?

(a) daily before breakfast
(b) daily at night
(c) twice daily, night and morning
(d) monthly

6 Where should behaviour therapy charts be kept?

(a) in the office
(b) in the medical notes
(c) in the office and by Anne's bed
(d) by Anne's bed

7 Initially Anne should not be given large amounts of food. Which of the following is the most dangerous complication which occurs if large amounts are given?

(a) vomiting
(b) paralytic ileus
(c) gastric pain
(d) excessive diarrhoea

8 Which of the following best describes what the nurse should do if
   four days after admission Anne complains of constipation?

   (a) inform the Doctor
   (b) increase her fluid intake
   (c) give her two glycerine suppositories
   (d) give her some bran at breakfast

9 Eventually Anne's diet should build up to a certain amount of
   calories so that her weight will increase. Which of the following
   number of calories is approximately correct per day?

   (a) 3000–4000
   (b) 4000–5000
   (c) 5000–6000
   (d) 6000–7000

10 Which of the following constituents form the basis of a diet for
    weight increase?

    (a) proteins
    (b) carbohydrates
    (c) carbohydrates and proteins
    (d) carbohydrates and fats

11 Which of the following best describes how Anne's initial diet of
    approximately 1500 calories should be organised?

    (a) what Anne likes two hourly
    (b) a bland diet four hourly
    (c) what Anne likes four hourly
    (d) a bland diet two hourly

12 To build Anne's diet up to a maximum intake will take some
    time. Which of the following describes the approximate time
    required?

    (a) 48 hours
    (b) three days
    (c) seven days
    (d) twelve days

13 Which of the following best describes how a nurse should approach Anne with food, initially?

   (a) be firm and unrelenting
   (b) try to persuade Anne to eat, gently
   (c) force feed her
   (d) allow Anne to eat as much as she can

14 One morning Anne has put on 2 kg. What might be the cause of this?
   (a) she may be retaining fluid
   (b) this could be possible on such a diet
   (c) she may have secreted something on her person
   (d) (a) and (c)

15 Which one of the following methods of nursing care may be most advisable at mealtimes if Anne is very reluctant to eat and is suspected of having vomited secretly?

   (a) asking a nurse to sit with her until one hour after she has finished her meal
   (b) ask all the ward team to observe her closely both during and after mealtimes
   (c) ask a nurse to sit with her during her meals
   (d) feed Anne slowly

16 On a behavioural regime which of the following weights should a patient gain a week on average?

   (a) 1.5 kg
   (b) 2 kg
   (c) 2.5 kg
   (d) 3 kg

17 Which is the most important reason why Chlorpromazine is sometimes given to anorexic patients before mealtimes?

   (a) to reduce anxiety and restlessness
   (b) it is an appetite stimulant
   (c) it is rapidly absorbed before mealtimes
   (d) (a), (b) and (c)

18 The psychiatrist decides that Anne's parents need to have some psychotherapy to explore their feelings as he thinks that they may have contributed to Anne's illness. Who of the following may be the most appropriate person to do such work?

(a) the consultant who sees Anne weekly and has a close therapeutic relationship with her
(b) the registrar who is not directly involved with Anne
(c) the ward sister who has planned Anne's care
(d) the senior house officer who gets on very well with Anne on a superficial level

19 Which would be the most advisable course of action when Anne has reached her target weight?

(a) to send her home
(b) gradually reduce her diet to a normal level
(c) begin intensive psychotherapy
(d) discuss her sexuality with her

20 Which of the following statements best describes the advice a nurse would give Anne and her mother regarding how often she should be weighed after discharge. To weigh Anne

(a) daily
(b) weekly
(c) monthly
(d) not at all

Alcoholism

Mrs Barwood has been admitted to your ward for detoxification from alcohol. She is a thirty-six year old housewife, with two children of school age. Her father died of cirrhosis of the liver. Her husband is a business man and leaves her alone for long periods of time while he is in the Far East. She has no financial worries and gets very bored at home. Prior to marriage she worked full time as a florist.

She has come into hospital after visiting her general practitioner and asking for help.

On admission her temperature, pulse and blood pressure are within normal limits. Nothing abnormal has been detected in her urine. The doctor has prescribed a drug regime of Chlormethiazole.

1 Are the above paragraphs:

(a) a nursing assessment
(b) the nursing assessment of Mrs Barwood on admission
(c) a nursing history
(d) a medical history

2 Mrs Barwood's father was an alcoholic. Is the incidence of alcoholism in children of alcoholics:

(a) more likely than in the general population
(b) less likely than in the general population
(c) more likely if the alcoholic parent was male
(d) less likely if the alcoholic parent was male

3 Is the incidence of alcoholism in women:

(a) twice as common as that of men
(b) half a common as that of men
(c) less than a quarter as common as that of men
(d) more than four times as common as that of men

4 For which of the following reasons is Mrs Barwood likely to have started drinking?

(a) boredom and depression
(b) loneliness and depression
(c) boredom and loneliness
(d) loneliness and anger

5 The doctor primarily prescribed Mrs Barwood Chlormethiazole during detoxification to:

(a) induce sleep and reduce anxiety
(b) reduce delirium and agitation
(c) reduce anxiety and nausea
(d) reduce nausea and induce sleep

6 The doctors feel that Mrs Barwood is likely to be successful in stopping drinking. What is the most likely reason for this opinion?

(a) Mrs Barwood has no financial worries
(b) Mrs Barwood was motivated to seek help
(c) Mrs Barwood is only thirty six
(d) Mrs Barwood has two children to consider

7 After forty-eight hours Mrs Barwood's temperature rises to 37.6° Centigrade. Which of the following should the nurses encourage Mrs Barwood to do and how often should they take her temperature?

(a) have a tepid bath; take her temperature after this
(b) have a tepid bath; take her temperature hourly
(c) drink extra fluids; take her temperature hourly
(d) drink extra fluids; take her temperature four hourly

8 Mrs Barwood tells you how bored and lonely she gets when her husband is away from home. Which of the following would be the best suggestion for you to make?

(a) that she gets a full time job
(b) that she gets a part time job
(c) that she tries to discuss this with her husband
(d) that she tells the doctor

9 Mrs Barwood tells you that she has heard that some alcoholics can drink in moderation. She asks you if this is true or not. Which of the following would you tell her?

(a) that it is not true
(b) that it is true
(c) that it is very common
(d) that it is very rare

10 When Mrs Barwood has successfully withdrawn from alcohol and is ready for discharge. Which of the following would be necessary?

(a) to organise an outpatients appointment with the psychiatrist
(b) for her to return regularly to the ward
(c) to organise a social worker to sort out her finances
(d) for a home help to be organised

Community Psychiatric Nursing—Mrs Colley

A community psychiatric nurse has been asked to visit Mrs Colley who is a 60 year old widow who has been visiting the general practitioner regularly, complaining of tiredness and loss of weight. Physical examination and tests have shown nothing abnormal.

1 How should the community psychiatric nurse let Mrs Colley
   know she is visiting?

   (a) just drop in and introduce herself
   (b) write her a letter introducing herself and asking if she can visit
   (c) write her a letter introducing herself and saying she will visit
       on a certain date
   (d) write and ask Mrs Colley when it would be convenient for her
       to call

2 She initially visits Mrs Colley, who appears neat and tidy but
   very flustered, on a Tuesday. Mrs Colley offers the community
   psychiatric nurse a cup of tea and then discovers she has no milk.
   She starts to cry. Which of the following would be the best action?

   (a) to listen to her
   (b) for the nurse to offer to go and get some milk
   (c) for the nurse to ask her if she would like to go and get some
       milk with her
   (d) to drink the tea without milk

3 As the conversation continues Mrs Colley explains that her husband always managed the finances and gave her a housekeeping
   allowance. Since he died she has managed to pay all the bills but
   has cut back on food and heat. She also explains that although she
   enjoys television she has sent it back because the rental and licence
   have become too expensive. Which of the following would be the
   best reply?

   (a) 'Would you like to tell me exactly how much money you have
       a week to spend?'
   (b) 'How much money do you have to spend a week?'
   (c) 'Have you any children who could help you with your
       finances?'
   (d) 'Would you like me to ask a social worker to visit?'

4 After some discussion it is established that Mrs Colley has sufficient finances for her needs. Which of the following would be the
   best action to take to help her?

   (a) ring up the television hire shop and have her television
       re-installed
   (b) together with Mrs Colley draw up a proposed plan of expend-
       iture including money for food, heat and a television
   (c) explain in detail how Mrs Colley could manage her money,
       drawing up a plan of expenditure for her to stick to
   (d) inform the general practitioner of her problems and ask him
       to help her

5 Mrs Colley says she feels much happier about everything now she
   has had a good talk. She would like the community psychiatric
   nurse to continue to visit her. The community psychiatric nurse
   agrees-when would it be best for her to return?

   (a) the following day
   (b) when she has had a chance to sort her finances out
   (c) at a time agreed by both of them, before the weekend
   (d) ask Mrs Colley to visit the nurse at the clinic the following
       week

Young man—Section 136

A young man is admitted to the ward under a Section 136. He has
been walking the streets with no shoes, talking to himself. He looks
unkept and rather unhappy.

1 Who must sign a Section 136?

   (a) a general practitioner
   (b) a general practitioner and a police constable
   (c) a police constable
   (d) a police constable and a social worker

2 Which of the following describes the terms of a Section 136?

   (a) a psychiatrist can rescind it at any time
   (b) it makes it possible to treat a patient
   (c) a person can be taken to a place of safety and then to a hospital
   (d) a patient can appeal against it

3 Which of the following would be a good idea if the patient is not too frightened?

    (a) to give him something to eat
    (b) to get him into bed immediately
    (c) to get his clothes and burn them
    (d) to introduce him to everyone on the ward

4 He wants to pass urine. He is asked to pass it into a jug as it needs to be tested. Which of the following is the most vital test to carry out on this man's urine?

    (a) acidity
    (b) drug screening
    (c) ketones
    (d) osmolarity

5 This young man agrees to having a bath and have his hair washed. When he undresses it is obvious that he has nits. Which one of the following lotions should be used to wash his hair?

    (a) gentian violet
    (b) gamma benzene hexachloride
    (c) benzidine
    (d) sodium citrate

6 Having de-infested him, the nurse is very concerned about his feet which are severely torn and oozing serous fluid on the soles. Which of the following is most important?

    (a) swabbing them for culture and sensitivity
    (b) covering them with a dry dressing
    (c) informing the doctor when he interviews him
    (d) putting him to bed so that he can rest them

7 Which of the following observations should be carried out on this man?

    (a) temperature, pulse and blood pressure
    (b) respirations
    (c) fluid balance, respiration and galvanic skin response
    (d) temperature, pulse, blood pressure, fluid balance and respirations

8 If this man has a temperature of 37.5°C. How often should this observation be repeated?

(a) 4 hourly
(b) 6 hourly
(c) 2 hourly
(d) hourly

9 The man agrees to go to bed after his bath. When he lies down he immediately sits up and says that he is too frightened to go to sleep. Which of the following would be the best way to deal with the situation.

(a) tell him not to worry and go to sleep
(b) say that you will sit by his bed and that he is safe
(c) ask him if he would like some medicine to help
(d) none of these

10 What is the most likely reason for the young man, shortly after settling in bed, telling the nurse that his name is Paul Mann? He has consistently refused to give his name before.

(a) he is frightened
(b) he has begun to trust you
(c) he feels a little more secure
(d) he has just remembered it

Mrs Smith—puerperal psychosis

Mrs Smith is a 30 year old woman who recently gave birth to her first baby, a son, James. She has been admitted informally with a diagnosis of puerperal psychosis. Mrs Smith appeared to be hallucinating as she said she could see water everywhere and expressed fears of drowning in it. Her 44 year old husband accompanied her and was very concerned and anxious about his wife. James was admitted with his mother because despite her illness she had managed to breast feed him.

1 In the first few days where should James sleep?

(a) in a single room with his mother
(b) in the nurses office
(c) in the ward
(d) alone in a single room

2 Which of the following would be the best nursing approach if, Mrs Smith frequently expresses her fears about seeing water that will drown her?

   (a) to disagree with her
   (b) to divert Mrs Smith's thoughts into reality
   (c) to discuss at length her fears and perception
   (d) to agree with her

3 Which of the following might it be advisable for the nurses to do for Mrs Smith initially, if she expresses great anxiety at looking after James even with supervision?

   (a) feed James
   (b) bath James
   (c) change James' nappy
   (d) put James in his cot

4 Which of the following would be the best course of action if the Doctors advise that Mrs Smith should have a good night's sleep with sedation? James is 14 days old and has been having a 2 a.m. feed.

   (a) to wake Mrs Smith at 2 a.m. to feed James
   (b) for James to stop his 2 a.m. feed
   (c) for Mrs Smith to express milk for the feed at 2 a.m. and the nurses to give it
   (d) for the nursing staff to give him a bottle of powdered milk

5 Mrs Smith picks up James and says she is going to take him home. The nurse is worried that she may harm herself. Which of the following should the nurse suggest Mrs Smith do?

   (a) go with James
   (b) go, if she left James behind
   (c) go, if her husband came to fetch her
   (d) remain in hospital

6 James has a bout of diarrhoea. His mother is on no sedation other than that at night. What is the most likely cause?

   (a) idiopathic
   (b) gastro-enteritis
   (c) ulcerative colitis
   (d) drug induced

7 What would the nurse do regarding James' diet if this diarrhoea did not persist?

   (a) add glucose water
   (b) feed him more frequently
   (c) change him to a bottle
   (d) leave it unchanged

8 Mrs Smith gradually improves and her husband is keen to have her home for the weekend with James. Who of the following would it be important to inform?

   (a) her general practitioner and midwife
   (b) her general practitioner, and health visitor
   (c) her general practitioner and community psychiatric nurse
   (d) all of these

9 Mrs Smith returns from leave, saying she has enjoyed herself. She shows no evidence of any delusionary or hallucinogenic processes. Which of the following should be written in the Kardex?

   (a) Mrs Smith is not deluded
   (b) Mrs Smith is not hallucinating
   (c) Mrs Smith is not deluded or hallucinated
   (d) there is no evidence of Mrs Smith being deluded or hallucinating

10 Which of the following would be the best nursing action if on the morning of discharge Mrs Smith bursts into tears and says that her husband is cruel and hates her?

   (a) tell her everything will be alright
   (b) insist she pulls herself together and goes home
   (c) listen to her
   (d) say that once she goes home, if anything happens to ring up the hospital

Mrs Reed–confusional state

Mrs Reed is admitted to your psychogeriatric ward from sheltered accommodation. She has become increasingly confused over the last two weeks.

Six years ago she was diagnosed as having carcinoma of the large bowel; she had a left hemicolectomy and has been well since. The doctors order a chest X-ray, and haemoglobin count. The lady develops offensive diarrhoea soon after admission; none of your other patients complains of this. After 48 hours her confusion has increased.

1 During your assessment of Mrs Reed which of the following would be the best description of her confusional state, given the above observations?

   (a) confusional state
   (b) dementia
   (c) confusional state of unknown origin
   (d) toxic confusional state

2 Mrs Reed's diarrhoea is quite severe. Which of the following nursing plans would be most appropriate?

   (a) fluids only
   (b) at least two litre of fluids daily
   (c) extra roughage in the form of bran
   (d) nil by mouth

3 Which of the following nursing actions may best help the problem of faecal incontinence if Mrs Reed finds using a bedpan or commode distressing?

   (a) place her in a bed near the bathroom
   (b) give her incontinence pads
   (c) ensure a nurse takes her to the toilet quickly when necessary
   (d) take her to the toilet four hourly

Miscellaneous

1 Owing to a patient recently being admitted it becomes necessary to move another patient's bed and locker. If there were four patients each with one of the following diagnoses which one would it be least advisable to move? The one with

   (a) simple schizophrenia
   (b) Korsakov syndrome
   (c) reactive depression
   (d) drug addiction

2 Mrs Smith is a 48 year old lady on your ward who is recovering from a depressive illness. She is described as having an extrovert personality. When planning activities for a Saturday afternoon which of the following would be best for Mrs Smith?

(a) a game of patience
(b) knitting
(c) reading a book
(d) going for a walk with a nurse and other patients

3 How should a nurse deal with the following situation? Mr Levi has been in hospital for several months since his wife's death, which caused him to be severely depressed. He is gradually recovering and would like to go to the Synagogue but he has no relatives who could take him. Should she:

(a) explain to him the difficulties of organising this
(b) telephone the local priest and ask him to help
(c) telephone the local Rabbi and ask him to help
(d) arrange for a taxi to take Mr Levi to the Synagogue

4 Every time Mrs Jones, a 74 year old lady with dementia is visited by her daughter she crys. Her daughter is getting very upset and says she will not visit if this continues. Which of the following would be the best nursing action to take regarding her daughter?

(a) listen to her
(b) agree with her
(c) say it is important she visits
(d) counsel her

5 Which would be the most appropriate reply for the nurse to make in the following situation: Carol is twenty-six, she has been successfully treated for drug addiction. Everytime she goes on weekend leave she steals from her stepfather. This upsets her mother and arguments always occur. Carol says, she never wants to go home again because of these arguments.

(a) 'You are rather old to keep going home anyway'
(b) 'Do the arguments make you feel unwelcome?'
(c) 'Carol, how do the arguments begin?'
(d) 'I left home much younger than you'

6 Mr Jones is 54. He became very depressed after losing his job. Since coming into hospital he has improved considerably and has been attending the industrial therapy unit regularly. One morning he says that he does not want to attend the unit anymore. Should the nurse

   (a) tell him it is up to him entirely
   (b) ask him if there is any reason for this
   (c) suggest he may be fed up and once he gets there he will feel better
   (d) ring the industrial therapy unit and find out if anything has occurred

7 Which of the following can Sarah Gloss eat if she is taking amitriptyline?

   (a) cheese and meat
   (b) meat and potatoes
   (c) cheese and milk
   (d) (a), (b) and (c)

8 Which of the following may best help a patient with Korsakov syndrome to remember where his bed is, if they are not normally labelled in the ward?

   (a) remind him frequently
   (b) label his bed clearly with his name
   (c) encourage him to have a photograph of his wife on his locker
   (d) place his bed near the office

9 Mr Johns has visited his wife every day since she was admitted two years ago with dementia, despite the fact that she no longer realises who he is. He has recently fractured his hip and is in the local general hospital. His ward sister rings the ward and asks if it would be possible for Mrs Johns to visit him as he has no other relatives. Should the nurse

   (a) explain to the ward sister how confused Mrs Johns is
   (b) suggest that as soon as he is well enough, he comes to visit Mrs Johns
   (c) assure her you will do everything possible to arrange this
   (d) explain that Mrs Johns really does not recognise her husband

10 Which of the following statements would be best if a sister orders
    15 pints of milk a day on a 30 bedded acute admission ward.
    There is never enough for coffee after supper. The patients
    complain about this at the ward meeting, pointing out that much
    of it is used at breakfast on cereal. Should she

    (a) state that half a pint of milk each a day should be enough
    (b) suggest she investigates the possibility of getting extra milk
    (c) ask them why they want coffee after supper
    (d) suggest that they try to be more economic with milk

11 Jane's main nursing problem is that despite having a regular
    menstrual cycle she never uses sanitary towels until after she
    starts menstruating and so gets into a terrible mess. She is being
    treated for simple schizophrenia. Which would be the most
    appropriate nursing action?

    (a) instruct her on how to use sanitary towels
    (b) explain why she should use sanitary towels
    (c) make a chart and point out when she is due to menstruate and
         give her a pad then
    (d) together, chart when she menstruates and remind her to use a
         pad before it commences

12 Which of the following would be the best nursing action with
    Jack? He is 74 and can no longer manage to 'wet shave' every
    morning without cutting himself due to Parkinsonian side effects
    from major tranquillisers. His medication cannot be altered.

    (a) show him how to use the ward's electric shaver
    (b) arrange for a nurse to shave him
    (c) encourage him to grow a beard
    (d) allow him to wet shave, giving him plasters as necessary

13 Mr Crew is 70 and has a depressive illness. His IQ is 60. He finds
    great difficulty in playing scrabble. Is this most likely to be due
    to:

    (a) his age and IQ
    (b) his IQ and illness
    (c) his illness and age
    (d) none of these

14 Mrs Jones is 54. She suffered a severe depressive illness after her husband's death. She lost her job in a chemist's shop as a result of this. Her mood improved considerably over the six weeks since her admission and the doctor informed her she could go home soon. Since this conversation she has become very apathetic, but not sad and is still sleeping well. Is this apathy probably due to:

(a) recurrence of her illness
(b) lack of motivation to go home
(c) institutionalisation
(d) prospective unemployment

15 John is twenty four and suffers from epilepsy. Which of the following features may lead you to believe that he is suffering from an hysterical fit?

(a) absence of corneal reflex
(b) incontinence
(c) response to painful stimuli
(d) unconsciousness

16 Mr Penny has been prescribed minor tranquillisers by the doctor. Which of the following is he most likely to be suffering from:

(a) schizophrenia
(b) endogenous depression
(c) mania
(d) anxiety

17 A schizophrenic patient Mr Watson refuses to take his medication because he says it is poisoned. Which of the following would be the best nursing action?

(a) agree that he need not take it
(b) give him his medication intramuscularly
(c) ask him if he would like to see you dispense it
(d) try getting him to take it later

18 Which of the following statements is true?

(a) hallucinations present in all psychotic illness
(b) insight is retained in all psychotic patients
(c) patients with psychotic illness may regress severely
(d) all psychotic patients are isolated

19 Is the main aim of the Health and Safety at Work Act of 1974 to:

(a) prevent cross infection in hospitals
(b) promote high standards of health and safety at work
(c) protect patients in hospital from dangerous objects
(d) ensure that no person works in excess of sixty hours a week

20 Nurses on a psychogeriatric ward have nowhere to store sani-chairs due to building works. Which of the following would be the most inadvisable sites to store them?

(a) in the bathroom
(b) by the patients' beds
(c) in front of the fire escape
(d) in the linen cupboard

21 A patient is described as an introvert. Which of the following statements defines this?

(a) a person who withdraws into himself and avoids other people
(b) a person who needs constant stimulation from others to be happy
(c) a person who is pre-occupied with social life and the external world
(d) a person who is sad, withdrawn and quiet

22 Which of the following actions should a nurse take if after doing a medicine round she has reason to believe that she gave a patient 100 mg of Chlorpromazine instead of the 50 mg prescribed.

(a) inform the nursing officer
(b) take the patient's blood pressure
(c) inform the patient's doctor
(d) take no action as the dose difference is small and probably safe

23 Which of the following amounts would be drawn up into a syringe from an ampoule containing 20 mg in 2 ml in order to give a patient a dose of 12.5 mg:

(a) 0.75 ml
(b) 1.00 ml
(c) 1.25 ml
(d) 1.75 ml

24 Which of the following nursing observations should be made first if a patient collapses suddenly. His:

    (a) blood pressure
    (b) temperature
    (c) pulse
    (d) colour

25 The first action a nurse should take when a patient becomes physically violent is to:

    (a) pysically restrain him
    (b) call for assistance
    (c) ensure no other patients are hurt
    (d) evacuate other patients from the area

26 Which of the following is an example of an 'open question'?

    (a) do you take sugar in your tea?
    (b) how do you like your tea?
    (c) do you think you are going to vomit?
    (d) do you want to vomit?

27 Which of the following people developed a 'pressure area' assessment scale?

    (a) Doreen Norton
    (b) Jean McFarlane
    (c) Nancy Roper
    (d) Sheila Quinn

James Grant—schizophrenia

James Grant is 26. He has been suffering with paranoid ideas about his neighbours. He has complained that they keep talking about him. Prior to admission he had called the police 'to sort his neighbours out'. The police found the neighbours quiet and friendly. James agreed to be admitted to hospital informally for a rest.

1 When assessing James he shouts at the nurse, telling her not to call
   him such awful names. In fact there is no evidence of anyone
   speaking in the area. Is he most likely to be suffering from:

   (a) an olfactory hallucination
   (b) a visual hallucination
   (c) a tactile hallucination
   (d) an auditory hallucination

2 James's temperature and blood pressure are within normal limits.
   However, his pulse is one hundred beats a minute. Is this most
   likely to be due to:

   (a) a bacterial infection
   (b) a state of anxiety
   (c) a cardiac disease
   (d) a viral infection

3 The doctors diagnose James as having a schizophrenic illness.
   Does this mean he is likely to be:

   (a) in touch with reality
   (b) out of touch with reality
   (c) completely aware of his illness
   (d) in complete control of himself

4 James tells a nurse that he is very frightened about the voices that
   he keeps hearing, talking about him. Would it be best for her to
   try to:

   (a) reinforce his fear
   (b) dispel his fear
   (c) deny his fear
   (d) understand his fear

5 James screams quite suddenly and then throws himself down in a
   chair, looking very frightened. Which of the following would be
   the best nursing approach to James?

   (a) firm and quiet
   (b) calm and quiet
   (c) loud and excited
   (d) quiet and excited

6 James commences Chlorpromazine tablets as prescribed by the doctor. He says that he would rather take medicine than pills. Would you:

(a) insist he takes the tablets
(b) ask him to take the tablets
(c) ask the Doctor to change the prescription of tablets to liquid
(d) omit James' Chlorpromazine at the medicine round

7 What should the nurse do if James finds the noise of the radio very distressing and there are several other patients on the ward who enjoy it.

(a) turn the radio off
(b) lower the radio volume
(c) take James into a quiet area
(d) ask James to tolerate other patients' needs

8 If James does not like washing and keeping himself clean what would be the best nursing action?

(a) for a nurse to bath James
(b) to give James a planned hygiene routine
(c) to leave James to wash when he likes
(d) to plan a hygiene routine together with James

9 James has responded to treatment over a period of six weeks. He is to be discharged, but to attend a day hospital. Is James most likely to attend the Day Hospital for:

(a) assessment and stimulation
(b) medical supervision and stimulation
(c) stimulation and socialisation
(d) observational stimulation

10 When James is due to be discharged from the ward, he asks to have the medication he is given explained to him. Should the nurse show him the written directions on the bottle and:

(a) tell him to read them at home
(b) sit down with him, and explain them
(c) explain them, using feedback to see that he understands
(d) get him to read them aloud to see he understands

Mrs Duff—manic depressive illness

Mrs Duff is admitted to a ward having been diagnosed as suffering from a severe 'manic depressive' illness.

1 Which of the following attitudes may best help while Mrs Duff is manic?

    (a) outgoing, open friendliness
    (b) an authoritarian manner
    (c) passive friendliness
    (d) quiet, firm manner

2 Which of the following is she likely to display while 'manic'?

    (a) delusions of poverty
    (b) delusions of grandeur
    (c) motor retardation
    (d) slowness of speech

3 Mrs Duff informs a nurse she has been taking medication for years but that it recently ran out. Was the medication most likely to be:

    (a) Lithium Carbonate
    (b) Depixol
    (c) Chlormethiazole
    (d) Diazepam

4 Which of the following would be the most appropriate nursing action if because of restlessness Mrs Duff would not sit down and eat a whole meal?

    (a) see that she gets adequate high calorie fluids such as milk
    (b) insist that she sits down and finishes a meal all at once
    (c) not worry over her intake at this stage
    (d) give her the left over meal later on

5 Mrs Duff becomes very excited at coffee time. She is not written up for any medication except night sedation. She says that she is going to knock the door down and leave. Which of the following people should the nurse contact for help first?

    (a) the nursing officer
    (b) Mrs Duff's consultant
    (c) the duty doctor
    (d) the security officer

6 Which of the following reasons is most likely to account for Mrs Duff becoming quiet and withdrawn 5 days after admission?

(a) she has exhausted herself
(b) she is becoming depressed
(c) she is ashamed of her previous behaviour
(d) she is missing her home

7 Which of the following nursing actions may be the most useful while Mrs Duff is quiet, sad and withdrawn?

(a) to leave her by herself
(b) to sit quietly with her
(c) to encourage her to join group activities
(d) to try and make her smile

8 After four weeks in hospital Mrs Duff is able to go home. Her mood is much more stable. She is given Lithium Carbonate to take home and an outpatients appointment. Which of the following would be the most important to explain to her?

(a) how to recognise features of her illness
(b) that the hospital has enjoyed having her and that she must return to outpatients
(c) the necessity of taking her medication and attending outpatients
(d) the necessity of continuing to take medication

5 Nursing Answers

Nursing Process

1 (a) This should include care of the physical, psychological, social and spiritual needs of the patient in an organised manner.
2 (c) Without a careful assessment, it is impossible to plan nursing care.

3 (d) Before planning another method of care re-assessment is necessary. If the original assessment is incorrect then nursing care prescribed is likely to be wrong also. It is important that the patient is involved in his own assessments even if he says he doesn't mind. If a patient understands reasons for care, particularly if he defines his problem he is more likely to be motivated to co-operate.

4 (c) It is always best to state an approximate amount of fluid intake required, two litres is an average amount over 24 hours. Making the statement 'She likes tea' explains to any nurse what she enjoys and hopefully this is what she (the nurse) will offer. As the nurse has an idea of the required intake she *should* offer drinks regularly.

5 (c) A whole shift is a long time to leave a nurse with a depressed patient without relieving her, especially a student. If no particular person is responsible there is a danger of everyone assuming the other person is aware of Mrs Griffin's whereabouts. To keep Mrs Griffin in her nightclothes is very punitive and deprives her of dignity.

6 (c) You cannot plan individualised care satisfactorily while using hospital clothes which are often ill fitting, especially womens' bras and mens' trousers. There is no evidence to suggest that a certain number of nurses are required. The important thing is that they are motivated!

7 (b)

8 (d) The morning is a long time to sit with such a patient. 'As long as you can manage' can be interpreted as a variety of times from one minute to the whole morning. (d) clearly defines the length of time expected of the nurse and ensures her of a feedback period. This period can be used by the senior nurse to teach, explain and motivate the nurse regarding Mrs O'Brien. Alternatively it can be used for the nurse to express her feelings about Mrs O'Brien.

9 (d) (a) is rather vague. (c) is a good answer but (d) is better in that it encourages Mr Bell to inform you whenever he feels dizzy.

10 (b) As accurate an account as possible.

Community Psychiatric Nursing

1 (b) (a) is not necessarily true, (c) not all hospital patients are institutionalised, (d) is not necessarily true.

2 (a) Often the nurse will find her attention is directed to a whole

family group. However, usually there is an identified patient who is referred to her.

3 (b) This would normally be a District Nurse's job. (a) and (d) are highly likely, (c) psychiatric nurses frequently regulate drug regimes of phenothiazines, long acting depot injections, and so on.

4 (c) Psychiatric nurses often get patients referred for the wrong reasons but it should be for their skills.

5 (b) Some services provide (a) and (c) but as yet not the majority. (See Reference [1] below.)

6 (b) (see Reference [2] below for a description of this).

7 (c) (see Reference [3] below).

8 (a) (see Reference [4] below).

9 (c) (see Reference [5] below).

10 (d) (a) is not necessarily true, (b) are true but the *most* important is (d) aiding individual care.

11 (b) It is very important to get a 'subjective' view of the problem from the patient. The patient cannot hope to partake in a treatment regime if his view of the problems have not been taken into account.

12 (c) The nurse should organise a review date when making the plan of care with the patient, which is mutually convenient.

References

[1] Sladden, Susan (1979). *Psychiatric Nursing in the Community, a study of a working situation.* Harlow: Churchill Livingstone.

[2] May, A. R. and Moore, S. (1954). *Report on Warlingham Park Hospital.*

[3] World Health Organisation (1975, March). *Working Group on the Role of Nursing in Psychiatric and Mental Health Care.* Saarbrucken: WHO.

[4] Carr, P. J., Butterworth, C. A. and Hodge, B. E. (1980). *Community Psychiatric Nursing.* (Table 3, page 27.) Harlow: Churchill Livingstone.

[5] Carr, P. J., Butterworth, C. A. and Hodge, B. E. (1980). *Community Psychiatric Nursing.* (Table 4, page 27.) Harlow: Churchill Livingstone.

Nursing with Reference to Sociology and Roles

1 (c) Physics is not a behavioural science.

2 (b) Relationships can be observed in behaviour, but do not consti-
   tute an answer in themselves.
3 (b) The essence is that his actions or behaviour are relevant to the
   role he is performing. (a) he is performing but his actions are
   observable which is not implied in this answer. (c) and (d) may be
   included in his actions but they are enough alone for a definition.
4 (c) Uniform can be reinforcing in that it identifies the nurse. If the
   'nurse's role' is to make the patient responsible for himself it may
   be inhibiting, in that it can be seen by a patient as authoritarian and
   he may become increasingly dependent on the nurse.
5 (b) Part of the psychologist's function is to measure ability of
   people's intelligence, memory, etc.
6 (c) This is a delicate surgical technique.
7 (a) Both psychiatrists and psychologists who have received analytical training can practice psychoanalysis.
8 (c) The midwife ceases to be responsible for a baby when it is 10
   days old.

Nursing Ethics

1 (b) (a) is not necessarily true. (See Reference [1] below.)
2 (a) (b) the patient may never accept responsibility if he is not
   motivated to take it. (c) this would not allow for patients to take
   self responsibility. (d) this is true but Answer (a) is best. (See
   Reference [1] below.)
3 (b) If there are procedures which are equally effective in eliminat-
   ing undesirable behaviour it is good ethical practice to restrict the
   use of punishment. Occasionally no alternative method may be
   available. (See Reference [1] below.)
4 (b) Honesty in dealing with colleagues is as important as dealing
   with patients. If the situation is already affecting her work it would
   be unfair to both her and her patients to leave the situation for two
   weeks.
5 (c) All the answers are important but not all safe care results in a
   response to treatment. Safe care should be good care and maintain
   a patient's dignity but the question emphasises 'safe care' thus the
   most relevant answer is 'no harm'. (See Reference [2] below.)
6 (a) This answer encompasses all the others. (See Reference [2]
   below.)
7 (c) (see Reference [3] below).
8 (c) This is a difficult situation. (b) nurse–patient relationships
   should be based on *trust* whenever possible. (a) there is rarely a

place for secrets in a theraputic nursing team, for example if you agreed to this and then a patient committed suicide you would be in an intolerable position. (d) may work but is not the best answer as you may be betraying trust.

References
[1] Butler, R. J. and Rosenthall, G. (1978). *Behaviour and Rehabilitation.* Bristol: John Wright and Son Ltd.
[2] Schurr, M. and Turner, Janet (1983). *Nursing—Image or Reality?* Sevenoaks: Hodder and Stoughton.
[3] *The Mental Health Act 1983.* London: Her Majesty's Stationery Office.

Mental Health Act 1983

1 (d)
2 (b)
3 (c)
4 (b)
5 (a)
6 (c) in England and Wales. (a) in Scotland
7 (d)
8 (d)
9 (c)
10 (c)

Brenda Tewson—attempted suicide

1 (c) To ensure she cannot harm herself.
2 (d) Rather than (a). In case an admission in the night needs close observation.
3 (c) She can then explain how she feels rather than you assume you know. As in (d) important to *sit*. (See Non-Verbal Communication, p. 16.)
4 (b) Less frightening for flatmates for her to phone. Better to give patient the responsibility rather than taking it oneself.

Electro-convulsive Therapy

1 (b)
2 (a)
3 (d) To cover themselves.

4 (c) (a), (b) and (d) are the responsibility of the anaesthetist and psychiatrist.
5 (b)
6 (b)
7 (a)

Mr Morgan—confusion

1 (a)
2 (b) Refer to Memory Section of Psychology, p. 11.
3 (b)
4 (b)

Mr Meredith—confusion

1 (d)
2 (b) He has not taken care of his nutrition for several days. His confusion may be caused by this or vice versa. Fluids are more essential than food.
3 (b) This includes provision for individualised care in a problem solving manner.
4 (a) N.B. (c) is not a nursing decision but a medical one.
5 (d) N.B. should include individualised nursing care.

Diabetes

1 (b)
2 (c)
3 (b) He is likely to go into a coma called *hyperglycaemic coma*.
4 (d) He has become *hypoglycaemic* and may rapidly go into coma if not given glucose.
5 (b)

Mrs Jones—agitated depression

1 (d)
2 (c) A single room can be very lonely. It is not advisable to place new patients with paranoid ones unless it is absolutely necessary.
3 (d) This is hopefully a small reassurance.
4 (d) It is too dangerous to keep them on the ward.
5 (c)

Miscellaneous

1 (c)
2 (c) Day care facilities cannot hope to observe 24 hours a day.
3 (a)
4 (a)
5 (b)
6 (b) Both (a) and (c) encourage regression.
7 (c) (d) may well be impossible and will increase the patient's dependence.
8 (b)

Anne Leak—weight loss

1 (c)
2 (a)
3 (b)
4 (b) Washing and toileting can then be used as rewards.
5 (a)
6 (c) So that she can observe her progress and one in the office so that if she alters her chart this can be monitored.
7 (b)
8 (a) Anne may be trying to induce diarrhoea, so get the doctor's advice. She may have a paralytic ileus.
9 (b)
10 (b) Too many fats can make patients feel very bilious.
11 (b) ⎫
12 (b) ⎭ This is in order to prevent paralytic ileus occurring.
13 (a) If Anne manages to manipulate the nurses initially it will be more difficult to get her to eat later in the programme.
14 (d) Sometimes fluid retention does occur. It is more likely that she has concealed a weight.
15 (a) It is much more difficult to induce vomiting after one hour, than immediately after a meal.
16 (a)
17 (d)
18 (b) Ideally the therapists for Anne's parents should not be hers too. Certainly not in isolation. However, if it becomes evident that the parents are ill or one of them is, there can be conflict in the caring role of the doctor or nurse who is looking after Anne.
19 (b) If she went straight home her weight may drop.
20 (b) You want to try and break her obsession about weight. So

daily is rather too frequent, monthly is rather too long as she could lose or gain weight dramatically in this time. Sometimes people with anorexia nervosa find it difficult to stop putting on weight once they have begun. Alternatively, as soon as they are discharged they stop eating.

Reference
Dally, P. & Gomez, J. with Isaccs, A. J. (1979). *Anorexia Nervosa.* London: Heinemann Medical Books.

Alcoholism

1 (b) (Refer to Nursing Process Section, p. 56).
  A full nursing assessment should include Mrs Barwood's opinions as well as the nurse's observations and account of her social history.
  Nursing histories refer to nursing care given in the past.
  Medical histories refer to medical care given in the past.
2 (a) (see Reference below).
3 (c) (see Reference below).
4 (c) The assessment given does not state that she is depressed or angry. Assumptions must not be made about individuals without knowledge.
5 (b) (a), (c) and (d) may result but the primary reason is (b).
6 (b) Unless alcoholics are motivated to stop drinking, success is almost impossible.
7 (d) This is not uncommon. Extra fluids should soon bring Mrs Barwood's temperature down. It is not necessary to take her temperature hourly.
8 (c) If Mrs Barwood can discuss this with her husband, possibly together they can find a solution. It is giving her both responsibility and independence rather than increasing dependence. You should not tell her what to do.
9 (d) This is an honest answer. It is always better to tell a patient the truth as nurse–patient relationships are built on trust.
10 (a) It is normal for patients to be seen again for assessment and support. If she is encouraged to return regularly to the ward she may become very dependent on it. Financially she does not require a social worker. A home help is not necessary.

Reference
Dally, P. (1982). *Psychology and Psychiatry*. 5th edn. Sevenoaks:
   Hodder and Stoughton. Page 127.

Community Psychiatric Nursing

1 (c) You need to introduce yourself. Turning up without warning
   may alarm her. If you offer a definite date she can always write and
   tell you it is not convenient. If you ask her when or if you can come
   she may not reply.
2 (a) You want to make a comprehensive assessment of Mrs Colley. (b), (c) and (d) will only focus on the tea/milk and not on her
   problems.
3 (a) This gives her a chance to refuse if she does not want to tell
   you. (b) gives her no such option. (c) if she does have children they
   haven't seemed to help so far; also, if possible, you want her to be
   independent. (d) it would be better to try and establish if there is
   any real need, or if Mrs Colley is deluded about money before
   doing this.
4 (b) Give Mrs Colley some independence and responsibility, allow
   her to have a say in how she manages her money.
5 (c) You want to give her responsibility in this decision but ensure
   before the weekend that she has some food in the house and is not
   in the cold.

Young man—Section 136

1 (c)
2 (a) A person can only go to one place of safety under the terms of
   a Section 136.
3 (a) He is a little dirty to put in bed. We have no right to burn his
   clothes. It would be kinder to introduce him to people when he
   has cleaned up.
4 (b) Drug screening is vital as he has a history of being on the
   streets.
5 (b)
6 (c) The doctor can then advise.
7 (d) Initially one needs to ensure that he does drink. The other
   observations are obviously vital.
8 (a) Should be sufficient.

9 (b) He has been very co-operative up until now, so this should reassure him.

10 (b) Probably not (a).

Mrs Smith—puerperal psychosis

1 (d) It may not be safe to leave him with his mother. The nurses, ward and office may be noisy.

2 (b) These thoughts are real to her but to agree may reinforce her psychosis. To disagree may frighten her.

3 (b) Due to her delusions and possible hallucinations about water.

4 (d)
(c) will be too much for Mrs Smith. In a psychiatric unit this would be difficult to manage aseptically.
(a) the Doctor wishes her to have a rest.
(b) it is far to early to stop a 2.00 a.m. feed.

5 (d) The nurse should not allow an informal patient to leave the hospital without informing the doctor. A nurse may detain a voluntary patient if she feels she is a danger to herself.

6 (a) The question does not state serious, so gastro-enteritis is unlikely.

7 (d)

8 (c) Health visitors rarely work at weekends. Midwives cease to be responsible 10 days after the birth of a baby.

9 (d) It should read 'There is no evidence of Mrs Smith being deluded or hallucinating'.

10 (c) It is important to listen and get as comprehensive a picture of her feelings as possible. She may be becoming ill again. (a), (b) and (d) do not allow her to express herself.

Mrs Reed—confusional state

1 (c) Assessment of this patient needs to be completed by the medical staff before a reason for the confusion can be established.

2 (b) To replace fluid loss. Normally (a) and (d) are at the request of the doctor.

3 (c) Incontinence pads will only help if she is incontinent not at the problem source. Four hourly toileting may not be frequent enough. Putting her in a bed by the bathroom may help but as she is confused (c) is the best answer.

Miscellaneous

1 (b) Refer to Memory Section in Psychology (p. 11). Patients with Korsakov syndrome lose 'short term' memory. If you keep moving their beds they may be confused and get into the wrong one.

2 (d) Refer to Personality section in Psychology (p. 5). Extrovert personalities like to be with other people. Mrs Smith is getting better so a walk with others would be preferable to a solitary occupation.

3 (c) A Rabbi is a Jewish leader. A Synagogue is a Jewish place of worship. (d) is a poor answer as he has been in hospital for a long time, it would be better for the Rabbi to help by either accompanying or organising for a Jewish hospital visitor to do so.

4 (d) Counselling is helping a person look at various possibilities regarding a problem, showing them alternative methods of dealing with the problem and allowing them to come to their own solution. (Refer to Communication Section, p. 16.)

5 (c) (a) and (d) are not constructive. (b) is giving Carol a suggestion that may not be correct, but which may be used in a manipulative manner. (c) may help Carol look objectively at the situation.

6 (b) (a) and (c) do not allow for him to explain how he feels. (d) this should be done if (b) fails. If anything dramatic had happened the Industrial Therapy Unit should have let you know.

7 (d) It is a tricyclic antidepressant.

8 (c) (a) and (d) will not help in the long term. (b) will help but if his is the only labelled bed other patients may tease him. However, as only short term memory is affected he should remember his wife's photograph.

9 (c) (d) does not matter if Mrs Johns does not recognise her husband as long as Mr Johns is reassured.

10 (b) (See Motivation Section in Psychology, p. 9). Half a pint of milk a day is not a lot if it includes that to be used on breakfast cereal. If patients have been sufficiently motivated to complain this should be taken seriously and encouraged. Patients become institutionalised and cease to complain if no notice is taken of them.

11 (d) Refer to Nursing Process Section, p. 56. Always include the patient when planning their care.

12 (a) Always encourage independence as much as possible. He can't be allowed to cut himself daily.

13 (b) It is unlikely that his age is a major contributing factor. An IQ of 60 is below average. (Refer to Intelligence Section, p. 3.)

14 (b) She probably has little motivation to go home as she has no job or husband. The hospital provides a secure, safe environment which could eventually result in institutionalisation.

15 (c) The other three features are usually only present in 'genuine' epileptic fits, response to painful stimuli is normally absent in a genuine fit.

16 (d)

17 (c) As Mr Watson is paranoid it is obvious that his medication is a necessary part of his treatment; delaying it is unlikely to be successful. The question does not state that the doctor has prescribed the medication intramuscularly. Sometimes suspicion is relieved in patients if they are shown the medication and allowed to see it dispensed from the bottle or jar.

18 (c)

19 (b)

20 (c) This would be very dangerous if a fire occurred.

21 (a) (Refer to Personality Section, p. 5).

22 (c) You must inform the doctor immediately if a drug mistake occurs. The Nursing Officer can then be informed.

23 (c)

24 (c) It is essential to establish whether a heartbeat is present because if it is not cardiac massage and artificial respiration must commence.

25 (b) It is imperative to get aid in case the situation becomes too difficult for one person to handle.

26 (b) This question cannot be answered by Yes or No.

27 (a)

James Grant—schizophrenia

1 (d)

2 (b) He is likely to be anxious or frightened.

3 (b)

4 (d) If you manage to understand it you may be able to dispel it.

5 (b) Excitement or noise may only frighten him more.

6 (c) When practising individualised care every effort should be made to assist a patient with such a request.

7 (c) Noise can be very distressing to people who are hallucinating.

8 (d) Whenever possible patients should be involved in formulating their care plans.

9 (b) (See questions on Day Hospitals, p. 42). A primary assessment will have been made at the in-patient unit.

10 (c) (See feedback questions in Communication Section, p. 20).

Mrs Duff—manic depressive illness

1 (d) An authoritarian attitude could result in her becoming aggressive. A firm, friendly attitude should give her some guidelines regarding her behaviour.

2 (b) All her activities are likely to be speeded up.

3 (a) This is the most likely drug for a person with a manic depressive illness.

4 (a) As long as she has enough fluids and calories to maintain her that is all that is required. This is necessary as she will be using a lot of calories due to her manic state.

5 (c) He can come and assess Mrs Duff and prescribe medication if necessary.

6 (b) Manic depressive illnesses are often cyclical. A depressive phase may immediately follow a manic phase.

7 (b) This shows her that you care for her. Group activities may excite her again after a severe manic episode. Asking or trying to make someone smile who is depressed is a very childish request.

8 (c) It is difficult to teach people to recognise features of a psychotic illness and cannot be done at the last minute. The necessity of taking her medication should have been explained previously but she should be reminded before departure.

References

The titles listed below are useful for reference and also for more general reading about psychiatric nursing.

Burr, J. (1981). *Nursing the Psychiatric Patient*, 4th rev. edn. J. Andrews. Eastbourne: Bailliere Tindall.

Koshy, K. T. (1982). *Revision Notes on Psychiatry*, 2nd edn. Sevenoaks: Hodder and Stoughton.

Prothier, Patricia (ed.) (1980). *Psychiatric Nursing—A Basic Text*. Boston: Little, Brown and Co.

Willis, J. (1979). *Lecture Notes on Psychiatry*. 5th edn. Oxford: Blackwell Scientific Publications.